MEDICAL BONDAGE

MEDICAL BONDAGE

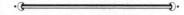

*Race, Gender, and the Origins of
American Gynecology*

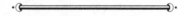

DEIRDRE COOPER OWENS

THE UNIVERSITY OF
GEORGIA PRESS
Athens

Paperback edition, 2018
© 2017 by the University of Georgia Press
Athens, Georgia 30602
www.ugapress.org
All rights reserved
Designed by Kaelin Chappell Broaddus
Set in 11/13.5 Fournier MT Std
by Graphic Composition, Inc.

Most University of Georgia Press titles are
available from popular e-book vendors.

Printed digitally

Library of Congress has cataloged the
hardcover edition of this book as follows:
Names: Cooper Owens, Deirdre Benia, 1972– author.
Title: Medical bondage : race, gender, and the origins of American gynecology /
Deirdre Cooper Owens.
Description: Athens : The University of Georgia Press, [2017] |
Includes bibliographical references and index.
Identification: LCCN 2017013982 | ISBN 9780820351353 (hardback : alk. paper) |
ISBN 9780820351346 (ebook)
Subjects: LCSH Gynecology—United States—History—19th century. |
Human experimentation in medicine—United States—History—19th century. |
Women slaves—Medical care—United States—History—19th century. |
Irish American women—Medical care—United States—History—19th century.
Classification: LCC RG67.U6 C66 2017 | DDC 174.2/8—dc23
LC record available at https://lccn.loc.gov/2017013982

Paperback ISBN 978-0-8203-5475-0

Dedicated to all the women in my family, past and present,
whose efforts have been unacknowledged and unappreciated.
Your lives and work inspire me.
Also, this book is for
Mary Cooper and Edward Bryan Cooper Owens—
thank you.

CONTENTS

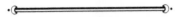

ILLUSTRATIONS

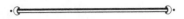

ACKNOWLEDGMENTS

Writing a book about women and men when you cannot hold conversations with them, observe their gesticulations, and look into their eyes is difficult. Yet writing books about subjects I am passionate about, interested in learning about, and inspired by is the reward for being a historian. I am overjoyed to produce a book that helps to place another piece of the puzzle on slavery and medicine together.

So many people, organizations, and institutions have supported me over the years. I am thankful for their assistance. I am indebted to the staff members at the following libraries for allowing me access to their records: the University Research Library at the University of California, Los Angeles; the South Caroliniana Library at the University of South Carolina; the University of Alabama Archives; the Reynolds-Finley Historical Library at University of Alabama at Birmingham (UAB); the Historical Society of Pennsylvania; the University of Pennsylvania's University Archives and Records Center; the Peabody Museum of Archaeology and Ethnology, Photographic Archives Collection, at Harvard University; the National Library of Medicine at the National Institutes of Health; the Library of Congress; the National Archives; and the American College of Obstetricians and Gynecologists (ACOG), now the American Congress of Obstetricians and Gynecologists. I spent nearly a month at the South Caroliniana Library, and Brian Cuthrell and Graham Duncan of the Manuscript Division were wonderfully attentive and helpful during my stay there. I owe a huge debt to Debra Scarborough, now retired from ACOG, for her professionalism, knowledge, support, and friendship. Debra introduced me to key texts on gynecological medicine, believed in my project from its inception, and located obscure sources for me. Mary Hyde, the senior director of the ACOG library, and her staff made my summer treks to Washington, D.C., pleasurable. Margaret (Peggy) Balch, of UAB's Reynolds-Finley, proved a godsend in the latter stages of my process.

I was fortunate to receive external funding from a number of institutions, including UCLA's Department of History, Center for the Study of Women, and Institute of American Cultures and the university's Ralph J. Bunche Center for African-American Studies. ACOG provided me with a generous and prestigious fellowship in 2007 that allowed me to gather much of the records I have on early gynecological medicine. Scholars at the University of Virginia's Carter G. Woodson's African-American and African Studies Institute selected me as a Postdoctoral fellow for 2008–9. I still consider my time spent at the institute as one of the most fulfilling professional experiences of my life. The University of Mississippi awarded me summer stipends in 2009 and 2010 that proved invaluable as I researched and wrote this book. The University of Limerick provided me a week's stay, when I was able to present my research to my colleagues in Ireland who helped me locate new sources for my work and provided critical feedback. Further, portions of an earlier draft of *Medical Bondage* appeared as "Perfecting the Degraded Body: Slavery, Irish-Immigration, and American Gynaecology," in *Power in History: From Medieval Ireland to the Post-Modern World*, edited by Anthony McElligott, Liam Chambers, Ciara Breathnach, and Catherine Lawless (Dublin: Irish Academic Press, 2011). Last, Queens College, CUNY, granted me a yearlong sabbatical during which I was able to finish this manuscript. I also received a William Stewart Travel Grant from the City University of New York in 2016 that allowed me to travel and present my research internationally.

Of course, scholars build their work because others have cleared a way for each successive generation. My mentors at Clark Atlanta University, Dr. Janice Sumler-Edmond and Dr. David F. Dorsey, transformed my life. Each good thing I accomplish as a historian is because of my interactions with and training from these two scholars. I am indebted to my dissertation advisor, Brenda Stevenson, whose expertise on U.S. slavery still impresses me. Ellen DuBois, Joel Braslow, and Caroline Streeter were wonderful dissertation committee members. While I was at UCLA, Jessica Wang, Scot Brown, William Marotti, Ra'anan Boustan, Valerie Matsumoto, Gary Nash, and Marion Olivas, former director of UCLA's National Center for History in the Schools, were most encouraging. My cohort members and fellow colleagues, Jakobi Williams, Miguel Chavez, Natalie Joy, Joshua Paddison, Jesse Schrier, Melanie Schmidt Arias, Stephanie Amerian, Mehera Gerardo, Sheila Gardette, Ebony Shaw, Lisa Boyd, Milo Alvarez, and Brandi Brimmer were wonderful colleagues. While in

Los Angeles, I was involved in the Southern California Alumnae Chapter of Bennett College, my undergraduate alma mater, and the sista-friends I made there sustained me in ways that still move me deeply. Marilyn Mackel, Diana White, and the late Marjorie Penalver loved on me deeply, and I appreciate their friendship. At UVA, Deborah McDowell and Claudrena Harold mentored me. I still stand in awe of their genius. My community of Woodson fellows is still intact, and I am grateful for it. While I worked at the University of Mississippi, I was a member of a welcoming and supportive community in the Department of History. Thank you. My colleagues at Queens College, CUNY, are smart, hardworking, and supportive. The editorial team at the University of Georgia Press has been amazing. Walter Biggins and Thomas Roche, thank you for serving as editors who wanted the best from me for this project. I would also like to thank the Race and Atlantic World Series editors, Richard Newman, Patrick Rael, and Manisha Sinh, for supporting my work.

Finally, I give thanks to my village, especially three recent ancestors who continue watch over me: Larry Norbert, Rodney Craig Goodwin, and Nakia Spriggs. Scholars of slavery, gender, and medicine Jim Downs, Sharla Fett, Edward Baptist, Jennifer Morgan, Barbara Krauthamer, Steven Stowe, Celia Naylor, Natasha Lightfoot, Catherine Clinton, Christopher Willoughby, Kellie Carter-Jackson, Natalie Leger, Dennis Tyler, Sonya Donaldson, Brandi Hughes, Nicole Ivy, Shennette Garrett-Scott, Cherisse Jones-Branch, and all those who have read and provided feedback on my work. My sista-scholar group members, Sasha Turner, Talitha LeFlouria, Kennetta Hammond-Perry, Lashawn Harris, and Sowandé Mustakeem, have literally been my greatest support system since I entered the profession. Thank you and I love you all dearly. Also, my sorors of Sigma Gamma Rho Sorority, Inc., have supported me since 1992. My family, my maternal grandparents, the late King Solomon Cooper and Mary Cooper, a retired black nurse—thank you for helping to raise me as a proud Low Country South Carolina Geechee girl. My paternal grandparents, the late Mr. Ben Cooper Sr. and Pastor Ella Bell Cooper, privileged their family and their faith, and I am grateful to have experienced their love of both. My parents, Arliree "Tee" Cooper and Ben Cooper Jr., along with my stepmother, Alveta, have always supported me, even when I decided at thirty years old to move across the country and start a doctoral program with a new husband. Thank you and I love you for telling me I was simply the best since birth; more brown girls need to hear and believe this message. My siblings and their spouses, Adrienne and Richard Putney and Ben Cooper III and Marquita Raley-Cooper, thank you for your unwavering support and love (plus, we literally share the best laughs together). My aunt Geneva Isa has been selfless with me since birth—thank you. My nephews Nicholas, London King, and the soon-to-be Paris Solomon: I do my work to prepare a legacy for you. Brooke Walker, you are my best friend and sister, thanks for the decades of love and support. Bryan, who knew nearly two decades ago that we would have experienced so much together? I am grateful for our journey, your gentleness, and your steadfast support of me. You have sacrificed so much to push me ahead unselfishly, often at your own expense. I love you.

MEDICAL BONDAGE

·❮━━━━━━━━━━━━━━━❯·

AMERICAN GYNECOLOGY
AND BLACK LIVES

> When invoking the term "body," we tend to think at first of its
> materiality—its composition as flesh and bone, its outline and contours,
> its outgrowth of nail and hair. But the body, as we well know, is never
> simply matter, for it is never divorced from perception and interpretation.
>
> —Carla Peterson, *Recovering the Black Female Body*

THE FIRST WOMEN'S HOSPITAL IN THE UNITED STATES WAS HOUSED ON
a small slave farm in Mount Meigs, Alabama, a lumber town about fifteen miles from Montgomery, a large slave-trading center. From 1844 to 1849,
Anarcha, Betsy, Lucy, and about nine other unidentified enslaved women and
girls lived and worked together in the slave hospital that Dr. James Marion Sims
founded for his training and for the surgical repair of his patients. He had his
workers, probably enslaved, build the hospital for the treatment of enslaved
women affected by vesico-vaginal fistulae, a common obstetrical condition that
caused incontinence, and that was brought on by trauma and by the vaginal
and anal tearing women suffered in childbirth. Years after he performed his
pioneering work, all experimental, Sims achieved success and an international
good reputation. He would later be known as the "Father of American Gynecology."

The women he operated on continued to perform the duties slaves were
expected to complete. These bondwomen tended to the domestic needs of the
Sims family, which included a sick child. They cooked, cleaned, stoked and
kept the fire burning during the winter, fetched well water, wiped sweaty brows

and dried crying eyes, planted and picked vegetables, and nursed their babies, all while serving at the same time as experimental patients. As Sims's surgical nurses, they learned the fundamentals of gynecological surgery from arguably the most successful gynecologist of the nineteenth century. During the five years they lived on Sims's farm, they helped him birth a new field. It is no exaggeration to state that these enslaved women knew more about the repair of obstetrical fistulae than most American doctors during the mid- to late 1840s.

In studies of James Marion Sims's career and especially of his "Alabama years," the occupational status of his enslaved patients as nurses has been consistently overshadowed by discussion of their illnesses. This study of slavery, race, and medicine, on the other hand, makes a sustained effort to examine and understand the richness of the personal and work lives of slaves, especially of Sims's slave nurses. Their experiences offer us a lesson about the relationship between the birth of American women's professional medicine and ontological blackness. During the antebellum era, most American doctors believed that blackness was not only the hue of a person's skin but also a racial category that taught substantive lessons about the biology of race and the so-called immutability of blackness. Following this biological theory, a black woman could be the same species as a white woman but also biologically distinct from and inferior to her. By examining the work lives of enslaved women patients and nurses through the prism of nineteenth-century racial formation theory, we can better understand not only the science of race but also the contradictions inherent in slavery and medicine that allowed an allegedly inferior racial group to perform professional labor requiring substantial intellectual ability.

In the case of Dr. Sims's slave nurses, scholarship has examined their exploitation as patients forced to work as surgical assistants. This book, however, shifts the focus to the lack of recognition these women received as nurses, even though nursing was considered a feminine profession in which intelligence and judgment were valued. This book also demonstrates how slavery and racial science were self-contradictory in their assumptions about black people's inferiority. Although historical records list the New York hospital Sims founded in 1855 as the country's first women's hospital, we also know that a decade earlier he had created an Alabama slave hospital for women. During its last two years under Sims's leadership, he taught his patients how to assist him during surgeries. Once Sims left the South for New York, he sold his women's hospital to a junior colleague, Nathan Bozeman, Sims's former medical assistant and a fellow slave owner, who continued operating it as a gynecological hospital and treated and experimented on patients from a primarily slave population.[1] Like Sims, Dr. Bozeman later sold the hospital and returned the enslaved patients to their owners. He went on to advance his burgeoning medical career and promote his button suture surgical method, which he touted as more successful than the Sims silk suture method.

For pioneering gynecological surgeons, black women remained flesh-and-blood contradictions, vital to their research yet dispensable once their bodies and labor were no longer required. Neither Sims nor other early American physicians viewed Sims's slave patients as the maternal counterparts to Sims in his role as the "Father of American Gynecology." There was no social or cultural impetus for professional white men, heavily invested in their racial, gendered, and slaveholding dominance, to do so. To remedy this failure to acknowledge their contribution, this book recognizes the unheralded work of those enslaved women recruited against their will for surgeries and made to work while hospitalized, and the labor of those poor immigrant women who willingly entered crowded hospitals in an effort to be healthy reproductively. *Medical Bondage* is not so much about historical recovery as it is about the holistic retrieval of owned women's lives outside the hospital bed. I place them in the annals of medical history alongside the doctors who performed surgeries on them.

Slavery forced sick women to experience their lives in ways unimaginable to other Americans. Slavery created an environment in which black women performed more rigorous labor than white women and some white men. Because the agricultural work that all enslaved people performed was identical, doctors sometimes erased gender distinctions when they assessed the physical strength and health of black women. White people believed that black women could sustain the brutal effects of corporal punishment such as whippings just as black men allegedly could. When these women fell ill, a physical state where most people are allowed to be weak, white society objectified and treated them as stronger medical "specimens." As a consequence, enslaved women vacillated between the state of victim and of agent.

The historical arc of American gynecology resembles other American histories in that it is triumphant. It is a polyphonic narrative that contains the voices of the elite and the downtrodden, and if studied closely, this history evidences how race, class, and gender influenced seemingly value-neutral fields like medicine. In works such as Sharla Fett's *Working Cures*, Marie Jenkins Schwartz's *Birthing a Slave*, and Deborah Kuhn McGregor's *From Midwives to Medicine*, enslaved women and Irish immigrant women emerge as historical actors worthy of examination. These scholars have rightly focused on sexual violence, reproduction, and the family, and *Medical Bondage* introduces both science and medicine into the discourse. By chronicling the lives of enslaved women, this book demonstrates that slavery, medicine, and science had a synergistic relationship. It departs from the work of Fett, Jenkins Schwartz, and Kuhn McGregor not only because it is a comparative study of black slave women,

Irish immigrant women, and white medical men. It also delves deeply into the creation of antebellum-era racial formation theories about blackness: the idea that race was biological and determined one's behavior, character, and culture.

Further, my study broadens the work of important historians of medicine like Todd Savitt who have focused on race and medicine but not examined the central role of slaves in the history of gynecology. Historians of race and medicine have recast different topics such as antebellum medical care, the health effects of emancipation, and late-nineteenth-century concerns about tuberculosis, race, and the city.[2] My work returns the discussion to the plantation while also examining how American gynecology developed.

Medical Bondage also builds on two significant arguments about the relationship between slavery and medicine. First, reproductive medicine was essential to the maintenance and success of southern slavery, especially during the antebellum era, when the largest migration and sale of black women occurred in the nation's young history. Doctors formed a cohort of elite white men whose work, especially their gynecological examinations of black women, affected the country's slave markets. Each slave sold was examined medically so that she could be priced. Second, southern doctors knew enslaved women's reproductive labor, which ranged from the treatment of gynecological illnesses to pregnancies, helped them to revolutionize professional women's medicine. Slave owners used these men's medical assessments to ascertain whether a woman would be an economically sound investment. Was she a fecund woman or infertile? Did she have a venereal disease that could infect others slaves on a farm or plantation? These questions mattered, and doctors provided the answers for buyers. Most pioneering surgeries such as ovariotomies (the removal of diseased ovaries) and cesarean section surgeries that occurred in American gynecological history happened during interactions between white southern doctors and their black slave patients.

As a comparative study, *Medical Bondage* analyzes the medical experiences and lives of Irish women during the antebellum era, in addition to those of slaves of African descent. This study does not consider the work lives of Irish immigrant women as maids, prostitutes, and factory workers in every aspect but focuses in particular on the medical impact that gynecology had on them. By the 1850s, the massive influx of recently arrived Europeans had become intertwined with modern American medicine. There has been little written about Irish women's reproductive medical lives, although many of these women experienced multiple pregnancies, like most American women of the antebellum era. This monograph shines a brighter light on the biomedical experiences of one of the largest groups of immigrant women in America during the age of slavery.

Poor Irish-born women relied disproportionately on hospitals and physicians in northern cities. In some urban areas, Catholic hospitals were founded to meet both the spiritual and the medical needs of Irish women. In cities such as New York, doctors relied on this patient group as subjects for exploratory gynecological surgeries in much the same way southern physicians did enslaved women, because these women were an accessible vulnerable population.

Within the crowded field of slavery studies and the growing genre of race and medical history, this book offers a different narrative about the history of American slavery, race, gender, and medicine. My research also proves that slavery and Irish immigration were intrinsically linked with the growth of modern American gynecology. Sims's work on Irish immigrant patients, especially his first New York patient, Mary Smith, evidences that he practiced a form of nineteenth-century medicine guided by the belief that elite white lives should be held in higher esteem than poor, foreign ones even while he relied on immigrant and black women's disorders to discover cures for the illnesses of all women. It reveals how nineteenth-century Americans' ideas about race, health, and status influenced how both patients and doctors thought of and interacted with each other before they entered sites of healing such as slave cabins, medical colleges, and hospitals. Racial formation theories were being created and debated just as women's professional medicine was developing. American medicine was moving from the periphery to the center in global Western medicine largely because of the innovative surgical work performed by gynecologists. Pioneering gynecological surgical procedures, many of which were initially performed on enslaved women and later on poor immigrant women, were responsible for much of the field's rapid advancement in cesarean sections, obstetrical fistulae repair, and ovariotomies. The import of these medical advances is immense because European medicine had previously dominated how physicians understood medicine in America. These theoretical and practical developments in women's medicine began to transform the United States into a leader in modern gynecology.

Up until the late eighteenth century, U.S. physicians relied on the ancient Greek and Roman humoral system of understanding and treating the body.[3] For example, American doctors, like their European colleagues, bled their patients to release toxins. The practice was a common one and was popularized by leading medical men such as early American patriot Benjamin Rush, who is now considered the "Father of American Medicine." Early on Rush also asserted that blackness was a genetic pathology and taught his medical students that blackness was a form of leprosy.[4] Although Rush's theory of blackness as a disease seems rooted in the Western world's general belief in scientific racism, he was asserting that black and white people were not different species. Thus blackness was not caused by natural anatomical differences, and ultimately black and white people were at least biologically identical.

American medicine came into its own after an American physician performed the modern world's first successful abdominal surgery and southern doctors began to use surgical methods that permanently repaired reproductive conditions. The reverberations of these surgical triumphs were felt globally. Following the publication of James Marion Sims's groundbreaking 1852 medical article on the treatment of vesico-vaginal fistulae repair, he received numerous invitations from European royalty to treat their female relatives for various gynecological conditions and diseases.

With Sims's achievement, American frontier medicine, much of it occurring in slave communities, had become a leading source for medical knowledge production globally. Yet the central role that enslaved women played in these advances—by providing doctors the bodies and sometimes labor needed for experimentation, treatment, and repair—went unacknowledged. Modern American gynecology could certainly exist without slavery, but slavery's existence allowed for the rapid development of this branch of medicine, and especially of gynecological surgery.

Like black enslaved women, Irish immigrant women faced a number of obstacles that obstructed their progress in society. These disadvantages included the debilitating physical effects of manual labor, sexual abuse, multiple births, disease, medical experimentation, and violence. My examination of the treatment of black and Irish women does not reduce them to uncomplicated victims of xenophobia and medical racism. I have chosen to follow theorist Saidiya Hartman's recommendation to not re-create the trauma and oppressive gaze that historical actors experienced at the time in my historical treatment of them. In my regulation of how "pained black bodies" are discussed and interpreted for readers' knowledge and ultimately their assessment, it is not my intention to cross the line of objectifying these historical actors.[5]

I direct attention toward not only enslaved women's lives but also those who were treated as "black" and bring into sharper focus what happened to them medically. My theorizations about their experiences, pains, uses, and their bodies should not be read as another way of reifying black women as disembodied "objects." Another challenge was locating sources where slave voices were not muted, filtered, or spoken by those who held power over them. I have attempted, however, to present these women as complicated, whole, and fully human, although the physical and psychological costs exacted by slavery were inhumane.

Since coining and defining the term "medical superbody," I have wrestled with its use because it is a fraught denominator.[6] Other than the problematic descriptor "degraded," which was broadly used to label disempowered women, no historic label from the antebellum era encapsulates the complexities and contradictions that were part and parcel of enslaved women's socio-medical experiences. Consequently, my use of medical superbody is intentionally messy, ambiguous, and contentious because black women's entrance into gynecology proved complex for white doctors, who viewed them through an optical microscope, using only two lenses, simplicity and complication. How could these women be both healthy and sick, strong yet rendered weak by the treatments and surgeries they endured? And ultimately, why were black bodies, which contained conflicting messages about their physical prowess and intellectual inferiority, positioned as the exemplars for pioneering gynecological surgical work that was to ultimately restore allegedly biologically superior white women to perfect health?

One of the more important functions of the "black" objectified medical superbody for white doctors was that black women were used not solely for healing and research but largely for the benefit of white women's reproductive health. They represented "the medicalization of life," whereby peculiar female diseases and even normal female biological functions were "problematized" and placed under the "advice procedures" of male experts who brought competencies within the orbit of an increasingly industrialized doctor-client relationship.[7] It was a space where the medical superbody was the "epitome of consumerism" and pedagogy.[8] "She" became "it," even in an arena like medicine, where patients were supposed to be treated as subjects, not objects. *Medical Bondage* is ultimately a historical telling of the impact of this medical scrutiny on the lives of enslaved women and poor immigrant women; it is also the story of the white medical men who fixated their gaze on these two groups.

Slave hospitals were the premier site for creating theories about black women's exceptionality, and medical journals were the ideal medium for describing what transpired in these hospitals and articulating the resultant notions. In their pages, doctors presented and defined black women as "the other." Medical journals allowed for the medicalization of black and Irish women that was critical to the racialization project and process.

Medical journals also described the "rival geographies" that existed between patients and early gynecologists.[9] In these spaces of respite—their homes, the woods, underground dwellings such as caves—slaves would use the time to heal themselves outside the surveillance of local whites and their owners. Slaves were almost always engaged in secretive activities, a necessity given the omnipresence of owners. Despite the furtiveness of slaves to "steal away," white doctors still had overwhelming access to black people's bodies and engaged in experimental gynecological work. White medical men moved black patients' bodies and body parts across a terrain that only they controlled. Historian Stephanie Camp has argued that "geographies of containment" were spaces where slaveholders put the idea of restraint into praxis. The slave hospital in this study is an exemplar of this kind of corporeal geographic containment.

Hospitals were the backdrops for physicians' medical writings that offered laypersons and professionals alike foundational texts that explained, usually in explicit and carefully crafted language, how to treat and think about black and white women patients who shared the same diseases. Medical journals were critical sites "where race was daily given shape."[10] These texts offered readers allegedly value-neutral explanations about black biological difference and disease. For example, women of African descent were believed to have elongated labia and low-hanging breasts and to be more lascivious than white women.[11]

Case narratives, the written descriptions of patient histories and exchanges with doctors, appeared in medical journal articles and chronicled the multifarious ways that black women experienced both antebellum professional medical care and racism. These sources are as important as plantation records, ledgers, and interviews in what they reveal about doctors' objectifying attitudes toward slaves and poor immigrants. Medical journals constitute the bulk of my source material. American doctors, especially pioneering southern ones who helped to create gynecology, saw themselves involved in a field that was becoming increasingly elite and professionalized and in some ways beginning to outpace European physicians' medical research in sexual surgery. Southern doctors believed "their medicine was inseparable from their need to pronounce it."[12] Contained within these doctors' writings are glimpses of slave life that are only beginning to gain recognition within the recent historiography of U.S. slavery.

Southern slave owners and medical doctors relied on these publications to manage their slaves. Slave management journals devoted the bulk of their pages to the medical care of enslaved people, especially women. Masters, mistresses, and overseers let physicians' published articles serve as guides for their treatment of bondwomen who were pregnant, had given birth, or suffered from gynecological ailments. Even as black women were sexually exploited and suffered from physical and psychological scars, often inflicted by the men who owned them, the maintenance of enslaved women's bodies was still considered a priority. White southerners knew black women literally carried the race and extended the existence of slavery in their wombs.

Medical Bondage attempts to repair the gaping fistula in the historiographies of slavery and medicine, just as nineteenth-century doctors did for their patients. However, in my effort to suture these historiographic holes, I humanize the experiences of the women who were both objects and subjects. The task is a difficult one because archives do not lend themselves to exploring and capturing the wholeness of enslaved people's lives. The study of U.S. slavery has changed greatly since early historian U. B. Phillips first wrote a pro-southern and Confederate-sympathizing history that praised slave owners for their benevolent treatment of their slaves. Since 1985, when Deborah Gray White and Jacqueline Jones inserted women into our discussions of U.S. slavery, historians have spent the next three decades examining enslaved women's labor, both productive and reproductive, and how the group resisted and negotiated their bondage. Since the late 1990s, a small number of scholars have investigated the impact of medicine (both professional and folk), healing, childbirth, and motherhood on enslaved women's lives.[13] *Medical Bondage* joins a small but growing cohort of scholarship that interweaves the histories of slavery and medicine to investigate how each system affected the other. Further, this book elucidates how reproduction made the experience of enslaved black women markedly different from that of enslaved men's. Enslaved women had more frequent contact with doctors and, due to gynecological problems, were placed in hospitals more often than enslaved men. They were the objects of study and fascination among white physicians.

The archival sources that allowed me to piece together the fragmented lives of women whose voices and experiences were published in snippets in the writings of white medical men are varied. I have relied largely on nineteenth-century medical journals, judicial cases from appellate courts, physicians' daybooks, the private diaries and plantation records of slave owners, census records, Works Progress Administration oral history interviews with former slaves, and slave memoirs. Other important sources that help to reveal the social conditions of the era are antebellum-era newspaper advertisements and medical texts and manuals. Fortunately, a number of archives have holdings devoted exclusively to slave history and medicine. In contrast, the bulk of archival records for Irish immigrant women's medical lives are scant, and most of my research on this group was culled from digital archives of nineteenth-century medical journals, medical textbooks, and hospital records.[14] Although the very earliest histories of slavery and medical history make no mention of enslaved women, they played a crucial role in the evolution of American medicine and must be acknowledged as scholars engage in the important work of tracing the origins of the intersections of race, gender, and medicine in early America.

This study also serves as a counternarrative to socio-medical histories that do not question the veracity of hagiographic top-down histories about "great white medical men."[15] Enslaved women played a central role in the advances made in gynecology by early pioneering gynecological surgeons, like Dr. Charles Atkins, who believed in the physical superiority of black women to bear pain easily. Atkins eventually published his findings about one of his slave patients, Nanny, nearly six years after her surgeries in 1825, in one of the country's leading medical journals. In medical journals, biological findings became ideology. Although southern white male physicians repeatedly encountered physically fragile enslaved women whose bodies were weakened by the rigors of harsh agricultural work performed in cotton, rice, tobacco, and sugarcane fields and multiple pregnancies, these men held fast to their belief in black women's physical strength and ease in childbirth.

Narrating the roles of enslaved women during the growth of nineteenth-century American women's medicine means that the history of American southern slavery must be understood in its entirety to tell a more factual story. Historian Ula Taylor reminds scholars who write about black women from our past to "speak to the silences" of their lives.[16] In order to combat the fictions doctors wrote about black women's bodies and their pain threshold in medical journal articles, it is important to home in on those moments when cracks in the narrative appear. For example, physicians described in their writings how and why they had to restrain their enslaved patients during childbirth and surgery. Why would this practice be necessary if black women were impervious to pain?

Earlier historians did not provide for the contextualization of slavery and gave scant attention to the examination of women, especially black women. In light of the contentious historiography that has emerged over slavery, race, and medicine, critical questions must be raised about the actual status of bond-women within the origins of modern American gynecology. Slave owners recognized the dangers, such as pregnancy and unsanitary work and living conditions, that affected slaves' lives and health. These men often shared "advice among masters" published in plantation management journals that discussed these matters at length.[17] Thus the history of black women's medical bodies was not created solely in medical journals but also by slaveholders who circulated "best practices" knowledge about black women and healing. For example, a South Carolina plantation owner advised other slaveholders to train enslaved women in the healing arts. He advised, "An intelligent woman will in a short time learn the use of medicine."[18] As a consequence, black women were drafted into medical practice, even if they did not want to heal others.

These enslaved women used healing to minister to their enslaved community. Faced with the possibility of life or death, soundness (good health) or sickness, infertility or barrenness, and professional acclaim or notoriety, black women executed a sophisticated "methodology of the oppressed" in their relationships with their physicians, owners, and communities.[19] U. B. Phillips, considered the first historian of North American slavery, detailed in *American Negro Slavery* how labor factored into black women's quotidian experience. Citing advice offered by slave masters, Phillips wrote, "The pregnant women are always to do some work up to the time of their confinement, if it is only walking into the field and staying there."[20] Former South Carolina slave Harry McMillan's recollections of enslaved women's network of care evidences the nuances of this methodology. McMillan noted that women "in the family way" performed the same work as male field hands. McMillan considered uninterrupted agricultural labor more important than providing care for enslaved women who had recently given birth, asserting that only "an old midwife . . . attended them. If a woman was taken in labor in the field some of her sisters would help her home and then come back to the field."[21]

Further, the work performed on enslaved and Irish women helped to legitimize this new branch of medicine. Like law, religion, and science, nineteenth-century medicine included many of the accouterments of racism that marked "black" bodies as inferior. They included the application of painful medical experimentations, without the use of anesthesia, even at a time when it was regularly used; separate and unequal medical treatment sites; and medical journals that racialized patients in their pages through idiomatic markers such as "robust," "strong," and "obstinate." "Black" bodies, and this term includes all bodies treated as black ones, were, as theorist Lars Schroeder notes, "written as agentless objects of white medicine."[22]

The men who practiced antebellum-era medicine needed bodies to advance the field and to recognize formal medicine as legitimate. Bodies, which served as clinical matter, were in high demand by doctors because most Americans treated themselves medically when they fell ill and rarely visited hospitals. Doctors dissected cadavers, performed surgeries on sick bodies and healthy ones; most importantly, they did so to heal their patients and gain knowledge. As medical fields branched off, gynecology, and to some degree obstetrics, emerged as one of the most innovative fields due to important surgical breakthroughs like the repair of vesico-vaginal fistulae, ovariotomies, and cesarean sections. Thus southern slavery was supported by the steady reproductive labor of enslaved women, and the reproductive and gynecologic illnesses of these women aided gynecology's growth. The ready availability of sick black female bodies did more than aid pioneering gynecological surgeons as they cured formerly incurable diseases. In the nineteenth century, the various medical interventions performed on enslaved women's bodies were the sine qua non of racialized medicine and the legitimization of medical branches like obstetrics and gynecology.

The historiography does not include texts that grapple with the complex positions these enslaved women occupied while under Sims's care. They learned to restrain patients while they were being cut with the surgeon's blade; they learned to cleanse and dress surgical wounds; they observed, over a five-year period, various reparative surgical techniques designed to remedy incontinence caused by obstetrical fistulae; and they did so under the watchful eye of a man who would become the country's leading gynecological surgeon. What did they do with this knowledge once Sims returned them to their owners?

Slave nurses were skilled laborers, and skilled slaves garnered more money for slave masters. Perhaps they became slave nurses or midwives after 1849, the year their experimentation ended. Unfortunately, the records are silent about their medical and personal lives once they departed Mount Meigs. Surely they must have integrated the medical knowledge they already possessed with the medical and surgical training they received as Dr. Sims's slave nurses. These women represent the intricacies of the antebellum slave South and the establishment of professional fields.

Like these historical subjects, this book highlights the complicated relationship between slavery and medicine. *Medical Bondage* is organized chronologically, but a common theme runs throughout it: the importance of enslaved women to the development of American gynecology.

Chapter 1, "The Birth of American Gynecology," contextualizes early American medicine with a particular focus on gynecology. Gynecology was not fully established as a formal branch of medicine until the 1870s. During its nascent period, however, slavery and enslaved patients were vital to the work that physicians performed to cure female ailments. A major theme that is examined is the confluence of racial ideologies about black people and antebellum-era medicine. As professional women's medicine grew in the 1800s, its ascendancy and legitimacy allow historians to also push past notions of continuity between how doctors treated all women in American society from its colonial beginnings to the antebellum era.

Chapter 2, "Black Women's Experiences in Slavery and Medicine," provides a historical examination of enslaved women's reproductive medical needs. The large number of enslaved women who needed reproductive care was one of the most significant boons to the outgrowth of gynecology. The institution of slavery allowed southern doctors to flourish professionally in what would later be called gynecological surgery. Due to the grueling work performed, the disproportionate number of sexual assaults enslaved women experienced, the unsanitary conditions of lying-in spaces, and inadequate diets lacking in vital nutrients and minerals, bondwomen were vulnerable to a host of diseases and conditions related to reproduction. This chapter explores how black women navigated their places in a rapidly growing medical field where white men eventually came to dominate a formerly all-female space for healing.

Chapter 3, "Contested Relations: Slavery, Sex, and Medicine," examines white southern male doctors' relationships with black female patients and the larger medical establishment. Many doctors believed in the distinctiveness of the South and acted out their roles as benevolent patriarchs not only on plantations but also in slave hospitals and southern medical colleges. Early pioneering doctors such as Joseph Mettauer, James Marion Sims, and Nathan Bozeman developed successful gynecologic surgical techniques because of their intimate knowledge of black women's bodies as patients and perhaps as sexual partners. They knew the black female body could serve as the medical exemplar for all women's bodies because there was no real physical difference in how black and white female bodies functioned. Yet they adhered to a racial etiquette that dovetailed with medical and scientific ideologies that espoused black biological difference. Further, these early gynecologists experienced gendered anxiety about their professional status and value as successful businessmen in an era when medical doctors were shedding their reputation as quacks and pill pushers.

Chapter 4, "Irish Immigrant Women and American Gynecology," describes the realities of poor Irish immigrant women's medical lives and demonstrates that their physical and medical experiences in sites of healing were similar to those of enslaved women. Through an examination of period newspapers, medical journal articles, physicians' notes, and hospital case records, I show how similarly these patients were written about, treated, and even experimented on by doctors who racialized their foreign-born patients. In this section I evidence what philosopher Frantz Fanon stated about the burden of race placed on the victims of racism (I substitute Irish for black): "Not only must the Irish woman be Irish; she must also be Irish in relation to the white man and woman."[23] Poor Irish immigrant women patients were also affected by racist thinking about their bodies just as enslaved women were. These women were marked because of their recent immigrant status and the racial tropes that defined them as aggressive, masculine, ugly, and physically strong women.

The last chapter, "Historical Black Superbodies and the Medical Gaze," delves into the ways that medical doctors conceived of blackness through a binary framework of sameness and difference. This chapter explains how the use of various categories of analyses such as race, gender, medicine, and class were fluid. Thus I employ a meaning-centered critical analysis rooted in the social, cultural, and political significance of the body. By doing so, I bring into sharper focus the lives of the enslaved and poor immigrant women. Further, the appropriated bodies of "black" women can also be understood through the daily spaces where antebellum-era conceptions of race took shape, in hospitals, homes, and slave cabins.

The history of American gynecology has always been narrated as a story about James Marion Sims's meteoric rise as the "Father of American Gynecology" during the antebellum era. Yet I argue in *Medical Bondage* that this origin story is more expansive and includes a larger set of historical actors who are also central to gynecology's birth: black slave women. Beginning with those nearly ten black bondwomen who labored under Sims as leased chattel, patients, and nurses, they serve as the counter to Sims's designation as "father." They are the rightful "mothers" of this branch of medicine. Yet patients do not leave archives; doctors do. For a slave-owning southern white doctor like Sims, however, black women were a ubiquitous presence, and they will remain pervasive in these pages.

Medical Bondage not only addresses the omissions but also revises the story of American gynecology's birth. I wrote this book as a response to the narrow binary categorizations of black slaves and white doctors in histories of medicine. It seemed that enslaved women in particular represented the only faces of oppression in studies about reproductive medicine. After I encountered the sources, which overwhelmingly pointed me to other marginalized women, in this case poor Irish immigrant women, I located a subject matter that complicated notions of "oppression" and "difference and sameness." I argue that studies of American slavery must grapple with all facets of slave life, including medicine, because every person born under the institution lived through a medical experience. The study of medical experiences provides a foundational framework for understanding the lives of the enslaved and, by extension, the oppressed.

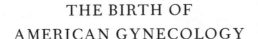

CHAPTER ONE

THE BIRTH OF
AMERICAN GYNECOLOGY

[Medicine] is a profession for which I have the utmost
contempt. There is no science in it. There is no honor
to be achieved in it; no reputation to be made.

—John Sims to his son, James Marion Sims,
the "Father of American Gynecology"

AFTER CONGRESS BANNED THE IMPORTATION OF AFRICAN-BORN SLAVES
in 1808, American slave owners became even more interested in increasing the number of slave births in the United States. At the same time that the
stature of the United States was rising globally, especially as an increasingly
profitable slave-based nation, another one of the country's industries, namely,
reproductive medicine, was developing and expanding rapidly. It was not long
before medical doctors and slave owners began to work closely to protect the
reproductive health of black women who were held in bondage. Doctors developed complex relationships with slave owners, slave traders, one another, and
finally, the enslaved women they treated for gynecological diseases. Despite
the complicated connections between white men and black women as doctors
and patients, they sometimes worked collectively in the name of healing, but
most often they did so separately. Their end goal was nevertheless the same:
to maintain the reproductive health of enslaved women so that they could continue to produce children.

Since the early seventeenth century, colonial Virginian legislators determined that the status of enslaved children would be tied solely to their mothers'

station.[1] A century later, bearing many children was a constructed measure of success for enslaved women, with some slave owners going as far as to reward slave mothers of large broods with gifts and, in rare instances, manumission. On Mary Reynolds's plantation, her owner promised to give every bondwoman who birthed twins in a year's time "a outfittin' of clothes for the twins and a double warm blanket."[2] Reynolds also told the story of a slave mother on her plantation who received certain privileges because of the sexual relationship she had with her master. A light-skinned enslaved woman, originally from Baton Rouge, Louisiana, was placed in a house, located some distance from the other slave quarters on the plantation. The woman had been bought as a seamstress, possibly a euphemism for "fancy girl" or sex slave.[3] After a few years, she bore a number of children for the plantation master, Mr. Kilpatrick. Yet he seemed so taken with his concubine that he violated racial etiquette and acknowledged his paternity of their children. According to Mary Reynolds, the plantation owner purchased the children's clothes, visited them daily, and allowed them to call him "Daddy" publicly. Of course, the archival records do not indicate how Kilpatrick's slave mistress felt as his concubine and the mother of his enslaved brood.

Unlike the fertile women Mary Reynolds mentioned who lived on her plantation, an infertile enslaved woman presented a problem not only for her owner but also for those white residents who lived in a slave society dependent on black women's reproductive labor. Alice Sewell remembered how her enslaved grandmother was "swapped away" because she "didn't bear children." She stated that after her grandmother had lived on the new slave farm, her current owner informed her former master "dat Grandmama was heavy with child." Sewell recalled how "sick" her grandmother's previous owner was over the sale and that Alice's mother never saw her mother again, "till she had all dem thirteen children."[4]

As black women's birthrates increased, white medical doctors began to work in midwifery in greater numbers too. Midwifery was not a medical field that men had previously controlled; it had been the domain of women for centuries. Since the country's colonization and founding, its citizens had believed that maintaining women's health was a job divinely ordained for women. Although there was a long history of male involvement in professional women's health care in Europe, American women—like most women globally—tended to one another when they gave birth. Despite women's predominance within the field, American doctors "masculinized" gynecological medicine by creating institutions and cultivating pedagogical approaches for men who would work exclusively on women's bodies.[5] These early Americans were building on a practice begun by their European predecessors nearly a century earlier. American men's entrance into this exclusively female terrain was regarded by some citizens as not only intrusive but also unnatural. Their outcry gained attention as the criticism entered the pages of colonial newspapers, like the *Virginia Gazette*, which described male midwives as "immoral" in a 1722 opinion piece.[6]

Despite these initial protests, however, white men continued to enter reproductive medicine over the course of the century. As a result, formally trained doctors devoted serious consideration to the complaints, conditions, and diseases of women. As these men became increasingly concerned with formalizing medicine more broadly and legitimizing certain branches of the field such as women's health, they transformed it into modern American gynecology. Most importantly, women's health improved globally as early American gynecologists innovated surgical procedures that aided in successful cesarean births, obstetrical fistulae repair (which stopped incontinence and repaired vaginal tearing after childbirth), and the removal of diseased ovaries via abdominal surgeries.

The partnerships formed by medical doctors and schools, especially those located in the South, with slave owners to treat the reproductive ailments that affected enslaved women gave them even greater access to black women's reproductive bodies and, later in the century in the North, to those of poor Irish immigrant women. Male midwives relied on the bodies of vulnerable populations like the enslaved and the poor to advance their medical research, to create effective surgical procedures to cure women of formerly incurable gynecological conditions, and, to a lesser degree, to provide a pedagogical model for physicians who were interested in understanding what they believed to be the biological differences between black and white women.

In slavery, healthy black people who labored diligently made the system economically valuable. Within the professional women's health-care world, deceased and living black women's bodies were also profitable. Doctors used the diseased reproductive organs of black cadavers to facilitate gynecological research and provide education in the field of gynecology. Career benefits also accrued to these medical men, who achieved their professional goals through the publication of their research in medical journals.

As the number of medical journals increased and they became more accessible, their popularity extended beyond the medical profession. Some lay planters relied on medical advice culled from these journals in the slave-management periodicals to which they subscribed.[7] Health problems proved to be a physical and economic burden to slave-owning southerners, and those who had a stake in maintaining a healthy slave labor force appreciated the availability of professionalized medical advice via the medical journal. Medical librarian Myrl Ebert, whose work provides the genealogy of American medical journals from 1797 to 1850, posits, "The advent of medical societies in America, combined with the need for better communication among native physicians, produced the first truly American medical periodical literature." Medical journals symbolized the growth of modern American medicine because they allowed doctors to make "demands for definitive ethics in practice, medical legislation for the protection of patient and physician, and the reorganization, expansion, and adjustment of medical education."[8]

If medical journals had by midcentury become so important culturally and socially, especially concerning matters of racial difference, how did this transformation occur so quickly when America had lagged behind Western Europe medically for nearly two centuries? During the late eighteenth century, American medical journals were limited and consisted typically of "reprints, translations, or imitations of European counterparts."[9] The *Medical Repository* began publication in 1797 as the first medical journal published in the United States, and in it a number of pioneering articles appeared. Dr. John Stearn wrote on the "use of ergot in childbirth" before American gynecology and obstetrics were even formalized as professionalized branches of medicine.[10] By 1850, American editors had published 249 periodicals about health and medicine, and out of that group, 189 were medical journals specifically. The growth of the American medical journal demonstrated that although Americans continued to rely on their kith and kin to care for them during illness, the status of formally trained medical men grew as they continued to professionalize and document their work through medical periodicals.[11] By the late 1870s, gynecologists' reputations had certainly improved from the low point indicated by the dismissive remarks made by the father of James Marion Sims at the start of Sims's career.[12]

In Augusta, Georgia, the brothers Dr. Henry F. and Dr. Robert Campbell served as editors of the Deep South's first medical journal, *Southern Medical and Surgical Journal*, and they served an exclusively slave population at the Jackson Street Hospital they founded. Enterprising and elite men like the Campbell brothers connected their private medical practices with other institutions such as slave hospitals, regional and national medical societies, and leading medical journals. In the case of the Campbells, slavery, medicine, and medical publishing formed a synergistic partnership in which southern medicine could emerge as regionally distinctive, at least through its representation in medical literature, and especially with regard to gynecology. For instance, Henry Campbell worked on enslaved patients as a gynecological surgeon, published medical case narratives of those operations in the *Southern Medical and Surgical Journal*, helped to found the American Gynecological Society in 1876, and in 1885 served as the president of the American Medical Association

(AMA).[13] For pioneering southern doctors like Henry and Robert Campbell, the American medical journal served to legitimize their careers as much as the work they performed in early American gynecology served to authenticate their professional writings.

Antebellum-era doctors wrote articles that were supposed to be value neutral and to be free of bias and prejudiced claims about patients' race, gender, and class. Much of their writing, however, reflected the scientific racism of the day. Gynecology, specifically, was becoming increasingly scientific because of its growing focus on research and experimentation. Gynecologists' ideas and practices demonstrated a broader belief that their forays into formal medicine should be trusted precisely because they were now leading a new medical field that was formerly the domain of women, who were considered inherently inferior. These doctors medicalized women's biological functions and problems that needed "expert" medical intervention. Moreover, their scientific research, which included experimental trials, accorded them the slowly growing respect of other Americans by midcentury.

Particularly by midcentury, physicians' medical writings offered laypersons and professionals alike foundational texts that modeled how to treat and think about black and white women and their perceived differences based on biology and race. The authors of these texts understood at the time, as historian Bruce Dain has argued, "that a sharp distinction between nineteenth-century biology and eighteenth-century natural history [was] not tenable."[14] Natural historians had primarily sought to classify and understand plants and animals, and they did so by describing the fertilization processes of plants and the mating of animals, for example, using language that likened them to human courtship rituals. In the nineteenth century, scientists and medical doctors began to not only study humans but also research ways to treat human diseases. The blending of science and medicine that occurred during the nineteenth century opened up space for research and even more rigid racial categorization to occur. Medical journals denoted this merger. Historian of slavery Walter Johnson describes medical journals as a site "where race was daily given shape."[15]

Racial reification occurred in these journals when questions emerged about whether certain diseases, features, and behaviors were endemic to women of African descent, for example, steatopygia (enlarged buttocks), elongated labia, low-hanging breasts, and lasciviousness.[16] The discourses on bondwomen and other racialized "inferior" bodies gave rise to the "black" female body serving as "a resource for metaphor," as literary theorist Hortense Spillers put it.[17] The descriptors in the American grammar book on race range from "Hottentot Venus" and "fancy girl" to "humble negro servitor." And one of the most common descriptive terms for enslaved black women was "breeder." In nineteenth-century America, the slave and, later in the century, the poor immigrant woman epitomized the "breeding woman," whose primary value lay in her ability to reproduce. There was little room for women who did not fit into this category. These names were all deeply rooted in America's long fascination with black women as hypersexual beings. Even as medical branches like gynecology and obstetrics grew, black women and those whom blackness was sometimes mapped onto, such as the Irish, were seen as willing and strong servants for white medical men, impervious to physical pain and unafraid of surgeries.

Southern hospitals that treated enslaved women who suffered from gynecological conditions proved to be critical sites where ideas about black and white biological distinctions were given credence. The Medical College of Georgia was one of the early sites of medical teaching about black and white differences. In mid-April 1850 in Augusta, Georgia, Mary, a twenty-eight-year-old married black woman who experienced irregular menstrual cycles and vaginal hemorrhaging, visited Dr. Paul Eve, a professor of surgery at the college, for treatment of her illnesses.[18] Eve was one of the South's leading surgeons and a founder of the AMA.[19] Besides disclosing her medical history and list of symptoms to the doctor (she had experienced problems with excessive vaginal discharge for three years), Mary also expressed concern because she had never conceived. Dr. Eve was not surprised by her symptoms; as he claimed, these kinds of gynecological ailments were common among local black women. He wrote, "The history of diseases among our negro population is generally very imperfect and unsatisfactory, and this is especially true as regards uterine derangements."[20] After diagnosing Mary with cancer, Eve assembled a surgical team, and they excised her cancerous uterus. The doctors claimed it was the first successful full uterine removal operation performed in the United States. Mary's postsurgery recovery was initially successful. As she recuperated, Mary asked the doctors a question that continued to nag her: why had she not yet menstruated after her surgery?

Mary may never have learned that the removal of her womb had rendered her infertile and not very valuable as a slave or perhaps as a wife who was supposed to birth children, for she died on July 22, 1850, three months after her initial visit to Eve. Her surgical team, however, understood fully the nature of her surgery and its likely consequences for an enslaved woman of childbearing age.

After Mary's death, her diseased uterus proved useful and valuable for another leading gynecologist, Dr. Charles Meigs, Dr. Eve's northern colleague. Eve granted Meigs permission to display Mary's preserved womb in his Philadelphia medical museum, so other doctors could observe how cancer ravaged uteri.[21] Even postmortem, some black women seemed unable to escape the gaze and ownership of white men.

Black women, like Mary, were exceptionalized in American society because of their blackness, alleged hypersexuality, and their seeming susceptibility to certain gynecological diseases. In reports of procedures performed on enslaved women, doctors used stark medical terminology that reduced black women's reproductive organs and bodies to mere "physical specimens." Their organs were used as clinical matter that was displayed for observation and dissection so that white women's pathologies and sick bodies could be cured. Although the biomedical research that nineteenth-century doctors conducted sought to locate the alleged biological differences between black and white people, white doctors used black women's bodies in their research because they knew that black women's sexual organs and genitalia were identical to white women's.

To be clear, male doctors viewed all women as inferior because they believed women to be neither as intellectually developed nor as physically strong as men. Medical doctors attributed all "women's complaints" to their "sensitive" natures, controlled by their uteri and nerves. Historian Londa Schiebinger found that for nineteenth-century American physicians, "females in general were considered a sexual subset of their race. . . . The male body remained the touchstone of human anatomy."[22] Black women were especially exceptionalized. Scientific theories and, later, medical ideas about their bodies, their fecundity, and their supposed abnormal ability to endure pain in childbirth can be traced back several centuries to the writings of European natural historians and male travelers who visited Africa. These ideas seeped into other areas too. White abolitionists throughout the British Atlantic world, who had aligned themselves on the side of black emancipation as early as the late eighteenth century, nonetheless accepted ideas that promoted black women as overtly sexual and much stronger than white women.

The purported differences that marked black women as distinctive took shape in the first exchanges between European men and African women.[23] In an early travel narrative, one author hypothesized about the sameness of West African men and women's bodies. He noted, "One cannot know a man from a woman but by their breasts, which in the most part be very foule and long, hanging down low like the udder of a goate."[24] These early male travelers were not always learned scientists and natural historians; nevertheless they carried their racialized narratives forward as the discipline developed. Natural scientists such as Carolus Linnaeus (Sweden), Johannes Blumenbach (Germany), Henri de Boulainvilliers (France), and Edward Long (England) ranked human beings using rubrics they believed were based in science and thus unbiased, and African people were nearly always ordered at or near the bottom of their scales. Linnaeus's seminal work on the origins of humankind, *Systema Naturae*, published in 1748; de Boulainvilliers's 1767 book on the theory of race and political conquest; and Long's *History of Jamaica*, published in 1774, all contained lengthy treatises on the racial inferiority of people of African descent. These publications represented, in the span of nearly two decades, how scientists' ideas of racial alterity and inferiority evolved from a belief in one's national origin as the sole indicator of racial difference to a conviction that human variation and hybridity were biologically grounded through the nerves, muscles, blood, and even bile of human beings.

Near the end of the eighteenth century, America's growing acceptance of scientific racism, or at the least a sort of proto-scientific racism, against people of African descent was highlighted by the publication of Thomas Jefferson's sole book, *Notes on the State of Virginia*. As a lay scientist, Jefferson established himself as one of America's earliest spokesmen on theories of race and nature, framing his ideas in the language of science. In Query 14 of his book, Jefferson defined the critical distinctions that, in his estimation, separated black people from what he thought of as less savage Indian people and the most highly evolved group, white people. Three of the most salient racial variances he observed among these groups were deeply embedded in western European definitions of beauty, respectable sexuality, and nature. The first difference Jefferson highlighted was the supposed ugliness of darker-complexioned African people when compared to the assumed beauty of lighter-skinned European people. The second mark of distinction concerned black people's temperaments. Jefferson noted that when black people were confronted with fear-inducing situations, "they [were] at least as brave, and more adventuresome" than white folks.[25] Per Jefferson's logic, black people's bravery stemmed from their childlike fearlessness and also their seeming naïveté about the perils of entering dangerous environments. Finally, Jefferson linked black women's perceived hypersexuality to the observable practice and scientific "fact" that African women preferred apes as their romantic and sexual partners rather than African men. Using matter-of-fact language, Jefferson asserted that African women had a "preference of the Oranootan . . . over those of [her] own species."[26] African people's physical traits—darkly hued skin, flat, wide noses, prognathism—were symptomatic of, Jefferson thought, their supposed primitive animalistic natures.

More broadly, this "biologically rooted racism," of which Jefferson was a proponent, further strengthened the anti-African racism of white Americans. Educated white people employed myriad methods to justify their belief in African inferiority and slavery. They wrote and decided court rulings that highlighted the "degraded" natures of black people in cases of rape, white ministers preached a Christian gospel that was proslavery, and men of medicine and science wrote voluminous accounts of the biological failings of black people as a degenerate race. Further, these racist ideologies influenced the burgeoning disciplines of biology and anthropology.[27] Yet, for all the measuring and experimenting this kind of racial formation theorization inspired, it failed as science because of its inconsistent findings.[28] As much as these conversations concerned the measurement of concepts like "nature" and "essence," what they did establish were significant attempts by white intellectuals to construct complex understandings of the seen and unseen biological forces of blackness such as wooly hair, thick lips, and even temperament. Under these circumstances, it is no wonder that nineteenth-century reproductive medicine emerged as one of the foremost fields in which the failures of race science were revealed. Once doctors examined, excised, and sometimes preserved black women's sexual organs in jars, how could they accurately detect whether a burst ovary or a small cervix belonged to a black woman or a white woman?

Several decades later, American scientific disciplines developed alongside British abolitionism and were translated into discourses on race and, later, the failures of both slavery and emancipation to properly civilize black people. By the mid-nineteenth century, famed abolitionist James Redpath even wrote that enslaved women [were] "gratified by the criminal advances of Saxons."[29] Thus notions of black women's innate inferiority worked in tandem with the tenets of racialized science. Like other branches of science, American reproductive medicine was influenced greatly by biologically rooted racism and was not a value-neutral field, despite how vehemently doctors asserted that the field was an objective one. Enslaved women were perfect medical subjects for gynecological experimentation because doctors deemed them biologically inferior to white women based on their research findings, yet black women supposedly had a high tolerance for pain. Also because of the low status of black women, white doctors felt no obligation to give merit to their thoughts on the matter.

Historian Deborah Kuhn McGregor has written about the tendency of early gynecologists to rely on emerging "scientific" methods to evaluate their patients, such as pelvimetry. This new tool was designed to aid doctors in assessing the size of a woman's pelvis and how easy or difficult the birthing process would be for the patient. Kuhn McGregor states, "Pelvimetry was also a tool of early physical anthropology. . . . The use of pelvimetry was profoundly embedded in perceptions of racial differences and went on to emphasize sexual differences and variation in the experiences of giving birth."[30] Few white Americans questioned the biases of formally trained medical doctors who authored articles that aided in the invention of a racialized metalanguage. Hence, what was thought to exist in the abstract could be made real because white medical doctors could prove through the "scientific" study of black people's "peculiar" diseases and behaviors that they were fit for slavery.

American gynecology's relationship to racial and gender prejudice was based on the precepts of an older Western, mainly Greek-derived *unani* medicine model that was used in cosmopolitan European medical centers for centuries. Historian Deborah Brunton notes, "In unani medicine, all women were believed to have a natural imbalance in their humors that made their constitution colder and wetter than men."[31] With a firm belief that women were literally the weaker sex, American doctors focused their attention on women's health. As a result, their published writings became much more focused on reproductive medicine. These publications signaled that the gynecological landscape had changed and midwifery was accorded less value. Gynecology, as a male-led profession, allowed doctors to determine that women's biological functions like libido, menstruation, and even childbirth were conditions that needed fixing. Since elite women tended to seek out the services of professionally trained doctors in cases of obstetrical emergency, medical men tended to publish more and more articles about abnormal births because those were the ones for which they were engaged.

Gynecology differed from midwifery in that men, not women, were delivering babies. During difficult births they used tools like forceps, and in rare instances, they administered anesthesia to women giving birth, though this practice was usually reserved for the most elite obstetrical patients. The following case highlights this latter point. In the country's earliest case of an American being given anesthesia to reduce delivery pains, Fanny Wadsworth Longfellow, wife of the famed poet Henry Wadsworth Longfellow, received anesthesia administered by a Boston dentist (dentists used pain-numbing medicines more frequently than other doctors).[32] Longfellow's example demonstrates how doctors privileged elite white women's alleged fragility and distress with physical pain.[33]

Medical doctors did not typically use anesthesia because of their well-founded fears that surgical patients could bleed to death in the time between unconsciousness and surgery. Dexterity and speed were much more highly valued than making a patient unconscious. For instance, in the case of James Marion Sims's experimental surgeries on slaves, Sims discussed in his memoir how he relied on speed in the surgical area to save his patients' lives.

More pertinent to men interested in medicine, especially southern men, was whether they could receive a quality medical education at their local medical colleges, if such an institution existed. Many southern men interested in women's medicine had to move away from home due to the dearth of medical schools in the region. In 1840 there were seven schools scattered throughout the South: the Kentucky School of Medicine, in Louisville (founded in 1817); in Virginia Winchester Medical College, in Winchester (1826), and Randolph

Macon College Medical Department, in Prince Edward Court House (1840); in Maryland the Washington University School of Medicine, in Baltimore (1827); the Medical College of the State of South Carolina, in Charleston (1832); and in Georgia Savannah Medical College (1838) and the Southern Botanico-Medical College, in Macon (1839). While many white southern men learned medicine through apprenticeships, some "sons of the South" traveled to leading European metropolitan centers like Edinburgh, London, and Paris for formal training in medicine. Those who remained in the United States tended to seek their medical educations in northern medical colleges. American medical college administrators offered students the following courses, which were typical of the course offerings in European schools: "1) anatomy, physiology, and pathology; 2) material medica, therapeutics, and pharmacy; 3) chemistry; 4) medical jurisprudence; 5) theory, and practice of medicine; 6) principles and practice of surgery; and 7) obstetrics and the diseases of women and children."[34]

Notwithstanding the small number of southern medical schools, the region represented an important site for pioneering innovations and achievements in gynecological medicine. Commenting on this issue, historian Joseph Waring emphasizes how vital black southerners, mainly the enslaved, were in this regard. Their sick bodies provided doctors with "great opportunities for the acquisition of anatomical knowledge."[35] And southern physicians carved out paths that guided their peers in how they treated and thought about their patients based on the patient's race and gender. Prominent medical men such as Ephraim McDowell (the "Father of the Ovariotomy"), John Peter Mettauer (the first American physician to perform a successful plastic surgery), François-Marie Prevost (the "Father of the Cesarean Section"), and James Marion Sims (the "Father of American Gynecology") revolutionized their fields.[36] They legitimized American medicine through their work in obstetrics and gynecology, and the larger Western world's medical researchers and their peers took notice of their work. Thus American slavery and early modern gynecology have intertwined roots that are distinctly southern. As much as white medical men are lauded for serving as the "fathers" of American gynecology, black women, especially those who were enslaved, can arguably be called the "mothers" of this branch of medicine because of the medical roles they played as patients, plantation nurses, and midwives. Their bodies enabled the research that yielded the data for white doctors to write medical articles about gynecological illnesses, pharmacology, treatments, and cures.

Pioneering medical men like Dr. James Marion Sims were heirs to a legacy left by a long line of older southern physicians and scientific researchers who relied on enslaved black bodies to find cures for ailments that afflicted all races. In a lesser-known medical case, President Thomas Jefferson began a smallpox vaccination experiment in 1801 that included both black and white members of his family and a few of his neighbors. Interestingly enough, Jefferson did not want white infants, some of whom were being nursed by vaccinated enslaved women, to possibly become infected with smallpox, especially if the experiment failed. So he ordered that only black babies would suckle from enslaved women.[37] A few years later, cesarean section surgery was pioneered in Louisiana solely on enslaved women by French-born surgeon François-Marie Prevost, who had repatriated to the southern state from Haiti after the Haitian revolution.

The professionalization of American medicine during the early nineteenth century culminated in the establishment of the AMA in 1847, and medical doctors' interest in establishing national reputations for themselves worked alongside their desire to build an institution. The antebellum era saw significant advances in gynecological research as gynecological surgeons first performed abdominal surgeries that removed diseased ovaries, delivered babies via cesarean section, and repaired vesico-vaginal fistulae, a common and non-life-threatening condition that affected many parturient teenaged girls and women.

Unlike ovariotomies and cesarean section surgeries, which required abdominal cutting, surgeries to correct vesico-vaginal or obstetrical fistulae entailed a low risk of death. Women lost little blood during fistula surgeries. During childbirth when vaginal tearing occurred, the woman's bladder (vesico-) became exposed because of the fistula (hole) formed while pushing the child out the birth canal. Once much of the upper vaginal tissue was sloughed away, an opening allowed for a "continuous involuntary discharge of urine into the vaginal vault."[38] Vesico-vaginal fistula patients suffered from incontinence, infections, and strong odors, and many became depressed. These women were quite often ostracized because of the stench that emanated from the constant stream of urine and sometimes feces that trickled from the fistula.

Because the future of slavery and the South's growing ascendancy as a global economic leader depended on black women's fecundity and the birth of their healthy slave offspring, southern doctors found no shortage of bondwomen to examine and treat for various gynecological ailments. They removed burst ovaries, sutured holes in bladders, delivered stillborn children, and excised tumors. Southern slave communities were so flush with sick bodies that James Marion Sims boasted, "There was never a time that I could not, at any day, have had a subject for operation."[39] Some enslaved women's illnesses were so severe that medical doctors were brought in to replace the plantation nurse who normally treated this group. The following 1811 medical case describes one such case.

During a summer afternoon, a parturient enslaved woman, some seven months along, attempted to climb a fence. She fell and "discharged from the uterus at least two pounds of blood." Her fellow slaves were ordered immediately to carry her into the big house. They struggled to pick her up but could not do so because of her girth and "dragged her into the kitchen . . . The blood marked her passage to the house." She fainted as soon as she reached the entry.[40] Dr. Thomas Wright noted that he was present when the accident happened. He wrote, "Her clothes were cut off immediately, her head supported, her hips raised while she laid on her back on the floor. . . . She was now raised upon some blankets that laid near her, and cloths wet with cold vinegar and water were constantly applied to the abdomen and labia. . . . I now directed ten grains of the Prussiate in milk. . . . The discharge entirely ceased. . . . Uterogestation was carried to its full time and the patient had a good labour."[41] After the entire ordeal, Wright estimated that the woman had lost a total of six pounds of blood.[42] Fortunately, he had saved the life of the hemorrhaging patient and her fetus, but his bedside manner and treatment reveal how negatively he thought of the bondwoman. Wright describes how he had the woman's clothes cut away so that she lay naked in front of other slaves who observed him as he patted her vagina to stem the bleeding. It was obvious that he did not regard her as a member of "the delicate sex."[43]

Wright's subsequent article that appeared in the *Baltimore Medical and Philosophical Lycaeum* would come to serve as a tool of nineteenth-century cultural production about blackness; the point of departure from whiteness expressed in art, intellectualism, and nationalism; and a basis of pedagogy for other early American obstetricians and physicians. A large body could be dragged, dumped on the floor, disrobed, and laid out for observation by a mixed slave community as a point of knowledge production. This disrespect belies the fact that doctors like Thomas Wright needed their black patients, as a means to learn about curing disease, much more than their black patients needed them. In the case just described, medical men would learn two important lessons. First, doctors would be instructed about providing care for parturient patients who experienced intrauterine bleeding. Second, and less explicitly, white medical men would be taught how to treat black women in particular medical spaces. Tellingly, the article included no messages about sympathetic gestures that might cater to enslaved women's needs. As historian Elaine Breslaw argues in her work about health care in early America, "white doctors were free to perform procedures on black women that would have been socially unacceptable to white women, at the minimum violating the standard of modesty."[44]

In the same article, Wright acknowledged how flummoxed he was when presented with the earlier case of a white woman patient he treated in 1809 for severe, protracted uterine bleeding following her pregnancy. The doctor was concerned because the young mother was still bleeding heavily two weeks after she had given birth. Wright noted in his article that she was a "lady of a delicate constitution."[45] Afraid that she was too fragile to be helped, the doctor consulted with local colleagues. He was informed that an old midwife, who had treated obstetrical cases for forty years, used a digestible powder known as "Prussian blue" on her patients with great success.[46] The doctor was ready to test the effectiveness of "Prussian blue" but first had to investigate the character of the midwife. After a male colleague verified the midwife's credentials and character, Wright was satisfied that he could use her concoction to treat his fragile white patient and ironically, later, his "negro" patients.[47] The irony lies in the fact that Wright's experimentation on his white patient taught him how to treat the bondwoman, a reversal of the roles for black and white patients.

Wright was only one of countless white physicians whose medical work symbolized the dynamism of antebellum-era notions of race. As historian Marli Weiner has noted, white southerners' notions of racial and sexual distinctions between black and white people were rooted in an older "argument about superiority and inferiority. . . . Race and sex differences had to be understood in some manner that suited the ideological needs of a slave society."[48] Black people were alleged to be biologically distinct from and inferior to white people. This belief, however, had to be put aside when medical work was performed. Southern white physicians knew all too well that a black woman's vagina and cervix were identical to the vagina and cervix of a white woman. Thus the gynecological operations were the same for black and white patients, even if the bedside manner and medical treatment differed because of racism.

Southern doctors like Thomas Wright and his contemporaries stood at a crossroads where medicine and slavery converged in ways that continued to build on the era's notions of racial and gendered distinctions; paradoxically, their findings actually diverged from current nineteenth-century medical knowledge. Slavery's importance to their research could neither be denied nor ignored; it was at the heart of their practice and scholarship, even if these doctors did not explicitly identify the institution as the linchpin of their intellectual work. The presence of a black enslaved population that included enslaved women complicated conceptions based on black inferiority and women's fragility. How could these doctors explain, through their medical writings, that supposedly inferior black female bodies were being used to glean knowledge that was then applied to the treatment and cure of illness for superior white women? It was a perplexing question that many doctors avoided answering directly, largely remaining silent on the issue. Fortunately their publications, which included medical case narratives that outlined the gynecological illnesses of enslaved women, revealed the inconsistencies centered on race and biology in nineteenth-century medicine.

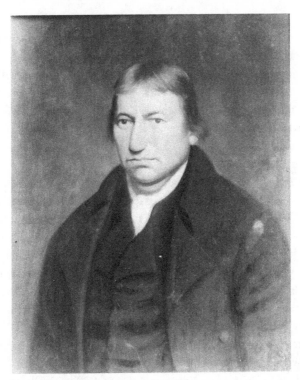

FIGURE I.I. Portrait of John Archer.
From the Collections of the University of Pennsylvania Archives.

As they were forging new paths in professional women's medicine, pioneering gynecological surgeons were also involved, sometimes quite heavily, in medical publishing. In 1768, Maryland-born John Archer became the first American granted a medical degree from the College of Philadelphia. Archer achieved some notoriety when he wrote about superfecundation, a rare occurrence in which two or more eggs are fertilized during the same ovulation cycle by sperm introduced through sexual acts with more than one male. Dr. Archer described two cases of superfecundation in his 1810 medical article, "Facts Illustrating a Disease Peculiar to the Female Children of Negro Slaves, and Observations, Showing that a White Woman by Intercourse with a White Man and a Negro, May Conceive Twins, One of Which Shall be White, and the Other a Mulatto; and that, Vice Versa, a Black Woman by Intercourse with a Negro and a White Man, May Conceive Twins, One of Which Shall be a Negro and the Other a Mulatto." In the article, the doctor detailed two interesting gynecological cases that involved pregnant enslaved women that had nothing to do with superfecundation. The first one concerned a thirty-nine-year-old enslaved obstetrical patient whom he had treated in 1783. The woman had experienced severe pain during her labor. After examining her, Archer observed that her vaginal opening was nearly closed because her labia were fused.[49] He did not identify the enslaved woman's birthplace, but it is quite plausible that this eighteenth-century parturient slave might have been born in West Africa in either 1743 or 1744, since the trans-Atlantic slave trade was thriving and not yet banned in 1783. If so, the woman could have had her clitoris and some part or all of her labia removed as a part of a rite-of-passage ceremony.

Archer operated on the enslaved woman, who belonged to "Mr. W.M.," with help from an enslaved midwife who had originally handled the obstetrical case.[50] The doctor "immediately introduced a director [guide] between the united labia and os pubis, and with a crooked bistoury, surgical knife with a curved blade." After this procedure, Archer "divided the labia . . . completely" opening the vaginal passage.[51] Archer's medical article documents one of the earliest cases of sexual surgeries performed on women of African descent in colonial British America; this kind of case would not be his last. In a discussion of a second case of fused labia, Dr. Archer describes how he treated a "young negro girl" who belonged to "Mrs. M'A."[52] Archer broke the parturient girl's fused labia with his fingers, and doing so allowed her to have a normal delivery despite the painful method employed.

Compared to Dr. Archer, Ephraim McDowell, a frontier doctor who would become lauded, some decades later, as the "Father of the Ovariotomy," is much better known in the history of medicine. His story exemplifies how challenging life could be for those who were innovators in the field of reproductive medicine. McDowell was born in the colony of Virginia in 1771. His father was a military officer and government official. When Ephraim was still a child, the McDowells relocated to Danville, Kentucky. As a young man, he entered the medical field, serving as an apprentice to a local medical doctor, but his apprenticeship ended abruptly after he was accused of grave robbing. He then left the country to study at the University of Edinburgh, arguably the premier medical school in the Western world.

After his stint in Edinburgh, McDowell returned to Kentucky, where he began treating the local community, which was mainly composed of white people and a smattering of black people. In 1809, Ephraim McDowell performed an ovariotomy on Jane Todd Crawford, a middle-aged white wife and mother. McDowell initially believed that Mrs. Crawford was experiencing a difficult pregnancy. After he discovered that she, in fact, had a tumor, he informed her that he would have to remove it surgically. Danville was a small town, and through the local grapevine word traveled quickly that McDowell planned to cut into the woman's abdomen to perform an ovariotomy. Surgeries

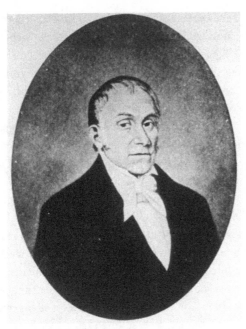

FIGURE 1.2. Portrait of Ephraim McDowell.
From National Library of Medicine,
http://ihm.nlm.nih.gov/images/B29869.

were exceedingly rare in the new nation, and in a frontier community like Danville, Kentucky, people believed correctly that abdominal surgery meant certain death for the patient. Some townsmen threatened McDowell physically because they believed the surgeon would surely kill Mrs. Crawford. Nonetheless, early on Christmas morning, McDowell removed Crawford's tumor, which weighed over twenty pounds. Amazingly, she survived and lived to be seventy-eight years old.

Dr. McDowell waited nearly a decade before he published the groundbreaking article that described his successful ovariotomy procedure, "Three Cases of Extirpation of Diseased Ovaria," in the *Eclectic Repertory and Analytic Review* in 1817. After the article's publication, McDowell was largely derided. European doctors were the most vocal in their criticism of him because American medicine was still in its infancy and static and had not produced trailblazing doctors. One of the leading critics, British surgeon James Johnson of the *London Medico-Chirurgical Review*, called McDowell a "backwoods Kentuckian." Johnson wrote, "All of the women operated upon in Kentucky, except one, were negresses . . . [and they] will bear cutting with nearly, if not quite, as much impunity as dogs and rabbits." He finally stated that as doctors, "our wonder

[was] lessened," since physicians understood that black women's propensity to handle pain was effortless.[53] In his hometown, too, McDowell did not escape the scathing rebuke of local slave owners who linked the doctor's unorthodox surgical work on Jane Todd Crawford with the episodes of grave robbing he had been associated with in the past. According to Mary Young Ridenbaugh, the doctor's granddaughter and biographer, "his own profession denounced him as a cruel, wicked person, who had no sympathy for man or woman—that he gloried in cutting open the belly of a woman."[54] She recalled how enslaved people responded to her grandfather's physical presence, writing: "The negroes of the village and the surrounding country being naturally ignorant and superstitious, whenever they spied Dr. McDowell walking in the distance, would rush into the nearest building, fearing that he might waylay and maltreat them. They feared him as they would some beast of prey."[55] The black residents had every reason to fear someone who appeared to experiment on black bodies with no real impunity despite the death of some of his black patients.

Despite the criticisms and fear he faced, McDowell continued to conduct experimental surgical work on women, but now almost all his patients were black. He found four black women who suffered from ovarian tumors in the local Danville area to experiment on over the course of nearly a decade, a stupefying accomplishment given Kentucky's small black population.[56] Gynecology was being formalized and legitimated on the reproductive organs and bodies of black women, yet in the literature doctors published, their bodies were not described as direct contributors to the growth of the new medical specialty. In nineteenth-century America, black women lived on the margins of society. Although black enslaved women represented a disproportionate number of the gynecological cases covered in medical journals, their inner lives remained peripheral in those publications. In their writings, doctors reduced the damaged reproductive organs and illnesses of slave patients to the knowledge they could provide for doctors.

The medical articles of Dr. John Peter Mettauer, another Virginian who became famous as a medical educator and pioneering gynecological surgeon, illustrate how early physicians wrote about enslaved women patients as objects. Mettauer was born into a prominent Prince Edward County slave-owning family in 1787. He followed in the footsteps of his father, who was a well-known surgeon. By the early 1800s, the county, located in the south-central part of the state, had transitioned from a struggling colonial outpost to a peaceful and prosperous area. The soil was fertile, tobacco was the major cash crop, and residents enjoyed successful trade relations, as the county was situated near the Appomattox River. A growing class of yeoman worked in the shops and small mills that dotted the country, and anchoring the economy was a flourishing

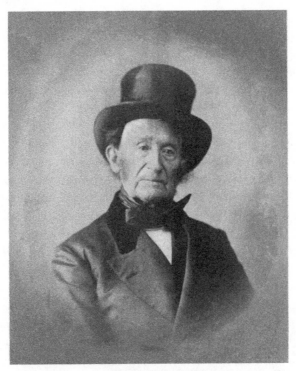

FIGURE 1.3. Portrait of John Peter Mettauer.
From George Ben Johnston, *A Sketch of Dr. John Peter Mettauer of Virginia:*
The President's Address to the American Surgical Association, July 5, 1905
(Philadelphia, 1905). Courtesy Historical Society of Pennsylvania.

slave system. Prince Edward County even boasted a free African American community, Israel Hill, named because it was their promised land like the one mentioned in the biblical story in Exodus. Unlike other southern counties, Prince Edward had a leading medical institute, and local residents welcomed the opening of the hospital that Mettauer founded there in 1837.[57]

Three years after he established his hospital, Dr. Mettauer performed one of the country's first successful vesico-vaginal fistula operations on a local white woman. Intellectually curious and ambitious, he performed experimental surgery on two additional local women to repair their obstetrical fistulae. One patient was a white woman and the other an enslaved woman. He successfully repaired the white woman's fistula but was unable to do so with the enslaved patient. During the following four years, Mettauer continued to perform experimental surgeries on the twenty-year-old bondwoman in an attempt to repair her fistula. Growing frustrated with his surgical failures, Mettauer blamed the enslaved woman for the persistence of her condition. He wrote that it was her active sexual life that kept her vaginal tears open and unhealed. Writing about the enslaved woman in an 1847 *American Journal of Medical Sciences* article, Mettauer stated, "The operation was repeated, but with no better success than the first. I continued, however, to repeat the operation twice a year, after the second trial, for eight times, and finally had to relinquish the case. . . . I believe this case . . . could have been cured in process of time, more especially, if sexual intercourse could have been prevented."[58] His language is both telling and jarring because he was so explicit in his description of the enslaved woman's sexual activity. Although his assessment is probably correct, Mettauer surely knew that enslaved black women had very little control over how their bodies were used sexually. In practice, Mettauer's slave patient had little or no agency to refuse men who wanted to engage in a sexual relationship with her, just as she could not end her participation in a gynecological clinical trial that proved ineffective for years. Mettauer's discussion of his enslaved patient in the *American Journal of Medical Sciences* obfuscated the grim reality that slave women faced regarding sex and their bodies. Perhaps unwittingly, he helped to legitimate another arena that was used to reify race for white Americans. His writing showed how American gynecology was being practiced and also how it was intellectualized in spaces like medical journals. Scholar Saidiya Hartman has theorized that "an inextricable link between racial formation and sexual subjection" was placed on black women in the nineteenth century.[59] And more specifically, Mettauer's narrative described the kinds of risks doctors and surgeons could and did encounter, as sexually active black slave patients served as physical encumbrances that could very much thwart their attempts at curing all women.

In spite of the challenges that Mettauer's enslaved patient faced, as a slave, a sexually active woman, and an experimental surgical patient, her medical example helped to unlock the mysteries that surrounded vesico-vaginal fistulae. Through his radical medical research, his creation of innovations such as lead sutures, and his surgical work in obstetrical fistulae repair, John Peter Mettauer designed a professional and intellectual realm for medical men who would follow in his footsteps.

Like Drs. McDowell and Mettauer before him, James Marion Sims was a southerner who advanced gynecology through his cutting-edge medical experimental work on enslaved women. Born in Lancaster County, South Carolina, in 1813, Sims came from humble beginnings. After finishing his undergraduate studies, he decided to attend Charleston Medical College. His father was contemptuous of his chosen field and stated that his son should be aware "there [was] no science in it . . . and no honor" that could be had.[60] Despite familial protests, Sims left the state to finish medical studies at Jefferson Medical Col-

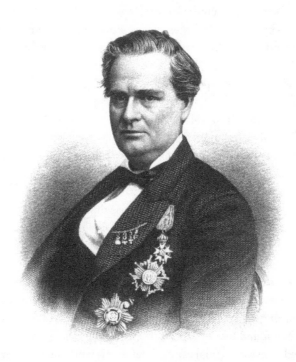

FIGURE 1.4. Engraving of James Marion Sims by R. O'Brien.
From National Library of Medicine,
http://ihm.nlm.nih.gov/images/B23841.

lege in Philadelphia.[61] After graduation, he returned to South Carolina to establish a medical practice. However, the deaths of two of his patients ruined his
professional reputation, and Sims relocated to Mount Meigs, Alabama. After
a few years in Alabama, he had become a well-respected doctor. Sims began
publishing articles about his medical work in the 1840s.

Dr. Sims was a prolific medical writer who published seven articles between
1844 and 1852.[62] His subjects ranged in scope from dentistry, to pediatric medicine, to general surgery, and finally to gynecology. They featured case narratives and illustrations of both his black enslaved and his white patients. By
the 1860s, Sims had become, arguably, the nineteenth century's most famous
gynecological surgeon; his experimental surgical work on enslaved women had
transformed the medical field. His reputation derived from the consistent positive outcomes he achieved based on the experimental gynecological work he
performed, quite an accomplishment for the era in which he lived. Many of his
peers could not duplicate successful surgical results during their clinical trials
and thus did not achieve the same level of fame that Sims possessed.

Like most men who entered gynecology during the first half of the century, Sims did so because of the urgent needs of women who suffered from a plethora of reproductive ailments. In his autobiography, he wrote about his initial distaste for gynecology: "If there was anything I hated, it was investigating the organs of the female pelvis."[63] Despite his "hatred" of female reproductive organs, however, Sims chose to perform a vaginal examination on one of his patients, Mrs. Merrill, who had been thrown from her horse. His examination revealed that she had a reversed uterus. Remembering a medical lecture he had attended in medical school, he opened Merrill's vaginal cavity wide enough so that the force of air pressure would help to pivot her womb to its correct position. It was literally at this moment that Sims was reminded of three enslaved patients who had earlier visited him because they suffered from vesico-vaginal fistulae. Sims was now convinced that if he could apply the technique he had used most recently on Mrs. Merrill on the three enslaved obstetrical fistula patients, he could cure them of their condition.

Sims wasted no time in testing his hypothesis. His first enslaved gynecological patient was Anarcha, a seventeen-year-old girl whom the doctor had first assisted during her protracted labor. During the two days she was under Sims's care, he had found that as a result of a difficult birthing process, Anarcha had developed a vesico-vaginal fistula.[64] Before his work on Mrs. Merrill, Sims had told Mr. Wescott, the teen's owner, "Anarcha has an affliction that unfits her for the duties required of a servant."[65] Sims also sent for Betsy and Lucy, who had visited him earlier because of their protracted labor, and leased them from their owners. As Sims later wrote in his memoir, he also "ransacked" the county and found "six or seven cases of vesico-vaginal fistula that had been hidden away for years in the country."[66]

Between 1844 and 1849, Sims experimented exclusively on enslaved women's bodies to aid him in locating the cure for this troublesome gynecological condition. In a speech he made before the New York Academy of Medicine, he explained how he had become a successful gynecologist. "Building a little hospital as a special field of experiment," he told his audience, "I readily got control of these cases, all of them healthy young negro women."[67] Commonly called a "sick house," the sort of "little hospital" that Sims described was an important component of the slave farm.

Antebellum-era physician James Ewell described the sick houses as a "cheap, coarse kind of building." He reasoned that good ones "ought to consist of but one large room, quite open to the top, well aired by doors and windows, and with a plank floor, that it may be frequently washed and kept perfectly clean."[68] Visitors to the South were fascinated by these slave hospitals and often wrote

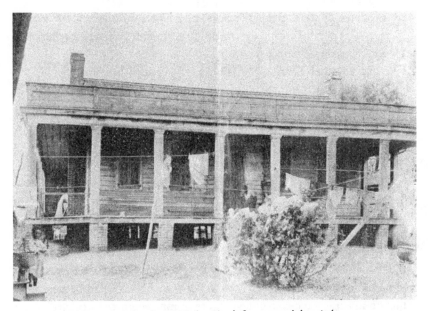

FIGURE 1.5. James Marion Sims's first women's hospital,
Montgomery, Alabama (1895), photographed by Edward Souchon.
Courtesy of the Reynolds Historical Library at the University of Alabama at Birmingham.

about them when they returned home. According to one such observer, Mr. Nordhoff, "The hospital at Hopeton [a South Carolina plantation] consisted of three wards. . . . One ward was for men, another for women, and the third for confinement cases. Although the women were allowed a month's rest in the hospital after the birth of their baby, they usually preferred their own homes, where they could gossip."[69]

Some slave owners took a dim view of sick houses. They urged fellow slave masters not to erect them, arguing that these facilities had a negative impact on the slave community. For example, Dr. John Douglass, a member of the South-Carolina Temperance Advocate, & c., warned that "sick houses or hospitals [were] unnecessary and injurious."[70] He feared that enslaved workers would become both melancholy and overly stimulated by the scenes of sickness from the hospital. Perhaps in Douglass's estimation, it was more fitting and natural for black enslaved nurses to be subjected to the sights of despair and illness among black people in the seclusion of slave cabins. White doctors, especially those who, like Douglass, cautioned against the introduction of sick houses, either did not consider or did not care that bondwomen resented the white male medical presence in their lives as much as the presence of a slave hospital. Despite the caveats offered by slave-owning doctors and planters, sick houses and lying-in rooms, spaces created for new mothers to recuperate, were becoming more common by the latter half of the 1850s.

The slave women's hospital that Dr. Sims had established proved indispensable to his research, for it allowed him to continue his experimental surgeries on "healthy young negro women." When, after two years, he had failed to cure any of these patients, however, Sims lost the support of the local white community, which included not only white residents who had observed his public surgeries but also the young white medical apprentices who had assisted him at the start of his experimental trials. (One of the latter was Nathan Bozeman, who later achieved fame in gynecological circles and criticized Sims's surgical methods for obstetrical fistulae.) After his white apprentices quit, Sims elected to train his enslaved patients to work as surgical nurses. The peculiarities of slavery meant that these women, all slaves whom Sims owned or had leased, would be trained as skilled medical workers, yet they would still have to labor as domestic and agricultural slave workers. It was a heavy double burden. Their situation illustrates the convoluted nature of nineteenth-century medicine in matters of race, class, gender, and status.

To more fully grasp the nuances of modern American gynecology's origins and expansion, one must consider the lived experiences of some of its first patients, enslaved women. Sims's patients suffered from a debilitating condition that, according to his description, made them "unfit" for the work bondwomen were to perform. Additionally, some of these women were forced to live far from their friends and family for the duration of the experiment. They raised children without the presence of fathers and nursed babies while also healing the scars they bore as experimental patients—and they did so even under the fog of postsurgery opiates that kept them dehydrated, constipated, and bound to their beds for at least two weeks while their bladders and vaginas healed. The women provided labor in the fields and inside the slave hospital that Sims had built for them. He created a rotational work and healing shift for his slave patients; while some women recuperated from surgery, the others labored on his slave farm, in his home, and in the hospital.

After five years of medical experimentation, Dr. Sims performed his thirtieth surgery on Anarcha and successfully repaired her fistula, closing it permanently with silver sutures, his improvement on John Peter Mettauer's lead sutures. Sims repeated the technique on his other vesico-vaginal fistula patients and cured them all of the condition.[71] They could now return to their former homes healed and hopefully be reunited with family and friends. From their slave masters' perspective, they had retained their value as breeding women who also now possessed a skill that could increase their owners' wealth, for they could possibly work as nurses who had trained under a renowned surgeon.

Following the successful conclusion of his five-year experiment, Sims returned his leased charges to their owners, and in 1852, he published "On the Treatment of Vesico-Vaginal Fistula" in the *American Journal of Medical Sciences*. Three years later, he moved to New York and opened the Women's Hospital of the State of New York. Thanks in large part to his experimentation on enslaved black women, Sims had established himself as one of the country's preeminent gynecological surgeons less than a decade after he began his gynecological career.

James Marion Sims's rise from obscurity to eminence followed a trajectory that other elite medical men had created for themselves for decades. Such doctors engaged in innovative experimental medicine; many relied on a disproportionately large population of enslaved women; and many published their findings in medical journals. The mid–nineteenth century was an era ripe for an enterprising and ambitious white man to ascend. Sims responded to the political climate of the 1850s by marketing himself as not only a doctor but also a medical entrepreneur. He named the position that vesico-vaginal fistula patients assumed during surgery the "Sims position," and he renamed the duckbilled speculum used to examine women's cervixes the "Sims speculum." The increasing ability of Dr. Sims and other men to heal and repair women's bodies encouraged the growth of gynecology as a profession and elevated it to a respected medical specialty. Their medical entrepreneurship also made them wealthy.[72]

In the mid–nineteenth century, men saw themselves as women's "protectors." Gynecology allowed them to enhance this role. Understanding the confluence of race and region is important because of the ways elite southern white men viewed their role as not only the protectors of women but also as "fathers." Many saw themselves as the "great white fathers" of their black slaves. Southern physicians who helped to advance the burgeoning field of nineteenth-century American gynecology also worked feverishly to maintain black women's ability to reproduce often and relatively safely. Thus the repair of any medical condition that could render an otherwise healthy slave woman incapable of bearing children further strengthened the institution of slavery. It was a system that valued enslaved women's wombs, the robustness of their sex lives, and ultimately, the number of children they bore, but it was also one that accorded black women neither respect nor wealth. Because male slave owners frequently sexually exploited the black women they owned, it is entirely conceivable that some doctors had sexual relations with the enslaved women they treated. Thus, many slave-owning physicians, and possibly James Marion Sims, not only served as the figurative fathers of reproductive medicine but also may have been the biological fathers of the enslaved children born during their experimental work in gynecology.

The demography of Sims's slave community illustrates how easily white men had access to black women's bodies. Sims owned and leased twelve females and five males on his farm. All the male slaves were young boys; in total the children ranged in age from two to twelve years old. Of the enslaved women on his farm, only seven or eight had reached childbearing age. Unlike the other slaves owned and leased by Sims, only one person was listed as a mulatto. An 1850 census described a one-year-old girl, the daughter of one of Dr. Sims's enslaved gynecological patients, as having a black mother and a white father. The little girl was the result of the reproductive labor her black mother performed as a slave and also possibly as Sims's gynecological patient and nursing assistant. Enslaved black women bore children for white men all the time, but birthing a child while they served as experimental gynecological patients was exceptional.[73]

Although a census record cannot prove the paternity of a slave child born to a white father, the child's existence gives rise to some critical questions about Dr. Sims's treatment of his enslaved patients. Was his enslaved patient impregnated against her will so that Sims could more easily locate a cure for her obstetrical fistula, since giving birth would reopen the woman's fistula? What other white men had access to this woman's body during her hospitalization and residency on Sims's slave farm? Sims detailed in his autobiography how members of the local white community withdrew their support for his experimental medical work. He suggested their lack of support occurred because of the repeated failures of his gynecological medical experiments. Could there have been another reason, perhaps one Sims did not want to address because of the ethical implications that would surround the birth of the mulatto girl on his slave farm?

Although these questions are speculative in nature, they should be considered serious inquiries about the nature of antebellum-era biomedical ethics and slavery. Although white Americans condemned and criminalized miscegenation, everyone knew that white men engaged in sexual relationships with black women as regularly as they had sex with white women. The presence of mulatto children revealed the hypocrisy of laws that banned interracial sex. Although the answers to these questions remain shrouded, Dr. Sims meteoric rise in the medical world demonstrates how he was still able to gain the trust of a community that had earlier rejected him. In 1848, four years after he began his experimental work, he was elected recording secretary of the Medical Association of Alabama. Nationally, Sims was elected and served as president of the AMA and the American Gynecologic Society decades later.[74]

Gynecological surgeons during the early and mid-nineteenth century were neither exceptionally cruel nor sadistic physicians who enjoyed butchering black women's bodies, as some scholars have argued.[75] They were elite white men who lived in an era when scientific racism flourished. Ideas about black inferiority were established and widely believed, as was the underlying assumption about black people's intelligence. Black women, particularly those who were enslaved, were a vulnerable population that doctors used because of easy accessibility to their bodies. Further, the value of black women's reproductive labor demanded that it be "fixed" when it was seen as "broken" by those who depended on their labor. As elite medical men like Dr. Sims met "the demands of clinical practice and those of clinical investigation," as medical historian Charles Rosenberg asserts, they were confronted with the challenges of experiencing lives that existed "between humanity and science."[76] This conundrum also included the enslaved, people who were regarded as human beings, chattel property, and clinical matter.

The medical notes and articles of white doctors who treated black women highlight the disdain they had for this group in sometimes unsettling language. The personal papers of a Delaware physician are graphic in their depiction of his handling of a black woman patient he reluctantly treated. In March 1853, Dr. William Darrach visited a black woman patient who lived "in a miserable hovel" over a canal. Her former physician had told Darrach that the patient was about to have an "abortion," which in the nineteenth century meant she was probably going to suffer a miscarriage. As Darrach approached her home, he heard the woman groaning loudly and miserably. He noted that he believed she was faking labor pains. Darrach chided her for her "deception" and left her with her child in the home. He returned "the next day . . . discovered [his] mistake and . . . found that instead of having an abortion she had dropsy."[77]

Black women patients had to navigate their relationships with doctors like Darrach, who detested their blackness and yet needed to repair their bodies. Despite the entrance of white men into gynecology and obstetrics, black women still found ways to provide medical care for themselves outside the gaze of their owners and plantation physicians. Investigating these women's successes and losses, especially in light of the pioneering medical research being conducted at the time, helps to uncover the hidden spaces within slavery. Moreover, understanding enslaved women's experiences in slavery and medicine can create a more comprehensive perspective about this group and their bondage.

·❦══════════════❦·

CHAPTER TWO

BLACK WOMEN'S EXPERIENCES
IN SLAVERY AND MEDICINE

She died 'bout three hours after I was born. . . .
They made my ma work too hard.

—Edward De Biuew, formerly enslaved man

D ECADES OUT OF SLAVERY, JULIA BROWN EXPLAINED TO GENEVA TONSILL,
an African American Works Progress Administration (WPA) interviewer, how her former owner practiced medicine on his slaves.[1] Brown recounted, "He'd try one medicine and if it didn't do no good he'd try another
until it did do good."[2] Brown's account illustrates the risky and experimental
nature of nineteenth-century American medicine. Further, the medical encounters she described also reveal the dimensions of slaves' powerlessness against
owners who took on the extra duty of caring medically for them. Julia Brown's
case is representative of that of any number of enslaved black women who were
rendered unable to heal themselves as they wished. The medical experiences
of Brown and other slave women symbolize the elasticity of early American
medicine, a field that integrated both formal and informal practices. Medical
doctors practiced medicine on black women's bodies as did slave owners who
formed close relationships with these medical men. Like trained physicians,
Brown's master risked killing his slaves in an effort to heal them. Julia Brown's
case illuminates how southern white men developed and deployed medical and
pharmaceutical methods that revealed how the value of black people's lives
shifted back and forth like the measurements on a sliding scale.

The growing body of literature on U.S. slavery and, more specifically, scholarship on the medical lives of enslaved people describe in great detail how valuable black women's reproductive labor was to both institutions. To birth a living and healthy black slave was rewarding for all members of slave communities including the mother, the plantation physician, and the slave owner. Each of these actors was invested in a slave child's birth for varied reasons. The investment in protecting the worth of black babies is well documented in the slave narratives of former bondmen and bondwomen who recalled how expectant mothers protected the children in their wombs while receiving the lash. There are numerous judicial cases across slaveholding states that reveal how vested owners were in the reproductive health of black mothers and their unborn children. Last, in murder trials that involved pregnant enslaved women as defendants, execution dates were halted until their children were born.

Arkansan Marie Hervey, who lived on the Hess plantation in Tennessee, remembered how parturient women on the plantation were punished physically. She stated, "They used to take pregnant women and dig a hole in the ground and jut their stomachs in it and whip them. They tried to do my grandma that way."[3] Had it not been for the efforts of her grandfather, who threatened those charged to whip his wife with violence, white plantation managers might have greatly harmed both mother and child. In an Alabama court case, *Athey v. Olive*, Littleton Olive bought a seemingly healthy pregnant slave, Matilda, from Henry Athey. Matilda's baby died shortly after the sale. Olive sued Athey for five hundred dollars on the grounds that Matilda was not of "sound mind" and also that Athey had breached their contract.[4] Surely Matilda experienced a tremendous amount of stress as she endured removal from her home to a new slave community, pregnancy, and possibly other factors that remain unknown. Further, her new owner blamed Matilda for producing a stillborn.

State of Missouri v. Celia, a slave stands as one of the most infamous antebellum-era criminal cases focusing on an enslaved woman's reproductive labor. The trial's outcome demonstrates that the judicial system prized the woman's pregnancy and unborn child rather than the teen mother who had been raped for five years by her late owner, Robert Newsome. Celia murdered Newsome, who had repeatedly raped her since she was fourteen years old. She had borne two of Newsome's children and was pregnant at the time of his death. The local court found her guilty and sentenced Celia to death. They delayed her execution, however, until she could give birth to her baby. As disparate as these two examples seem, they encapsulate the totalizing and punitive effects of the "maternal-fetal conflict."

Legal theorist Dorothy Roberts uses this term to describe the ways that laws, medical practices, and social policies differentiate between a pregnant woman's interests and those of her fetus. Roberts traces the genealogy of this conflict to slavery; of significance in her study are those cases where masters whipped enslaved women but shielded their bellies from the lash.[5] "Pleading the belly" was a process in English common law that allowed women in late-stage pregnancy to give birth before their death sentences were executed. Slave births created an incentive rooted in real property that merged with European religious and patriarchal notions that predated the institution of American slavery by centuries. Pregnant enslaved women lived in a society that invented and maintained practices that treated mother and child as separate entities. As a consequence, the mother's real value was in her reproductive health and her labor, which helps explain why reproductive medicine was so important during this era. White men with a stake in upholding slavery relied heavily on medical language and practices to treat and punish black women. Hence, slave owners and medical men upheld the practice of doing what they believed best medically to maintain a reproductively sound female slave labor force that was capable of breeding.[6]

The common linkage between the experiences of these enslaved women was their helplessness to resist the medical practices performed on their bodies. As much as enslaved women resisted their bondage and oppression, circumstances limited their power to defy their masters. Slavery and the antebellum-era medical field stripped slaves of agency at every turn, just as southern white babies suckled away the women's life-sustaining milk, a reproductive labor act that forced black mothers to provide calories for white infants' nourishment and growth at the expense of their own children's well-being. Slavery and the rise of American gynecology were the vessels that poured both life and death into black women's lives.

Although white medical men and many members of black communities expected these "manly" women or black "medical superbodies" to transcend fragility, many did not. The black female body was further hypersexualized, masculinized, and endowed with brute strength because medical science validated these ideologies. These myths led to the prevailing notion that enslaved women were impervious to pain. Tales abounded about black women's inability to feel physical pain. Delia Garlic recalled how shocked her mistress was when Delia fell unconsciousness after the mistress struck her atop the head with a piece of lumber. Delia stated, "I heard the mistess say to one of the girls, 'I thought her thick skull and cap of wool could take it better than that.'"[7] Former slave Harriet Jacobs shared in her memoir how her owner forced an enslaved woman to eat food that had killed his pet dog. The master did so because he believed that "the woman's stomach was stronger than the dog's."[8]

Further, the worries of bondwomen were rooted in the reality of the demanding physical labor they performed daily and the fear of the medical treatment they might receive as punishment. Edward De Biuew, who was formerly enslaved, suggested that his mother's premature death was caused by these factors. De Biuew remarked that his mother "died 'bout three hours after [he] was born" because "they made [her] work too hard."[9] William Lincrieux, an overseer who worked for Georgetown County, South Carolina, plantation owner Cleland Kinloch Huger wrote to his boss about how he continued to work two pregnant field hands who had tried to escape while laboring in Low Country rice paddies. On July 3, 1847, Lincrieux wrote that the parturient women were "confined which had done nothing in the hoeing of the Rice"; he made "no allowance . . . for sickness."[10] As much as enslaved women tried to resist their oppression, as the two parturient women had, they could do very little to protect themselves from the toll that field work took on their bodies. It is little wonder that enslaved women were at grave risk of suffering serious prenatal conditions. Prenatal risk was the price that slave owners, and by extension the doctors they hired to care for their female labor force, were willing to pay to ensure that black women continued to birth slaves with great frequency.

Motherhood was important to all women during the nineteenth century, but enslaved women's notions of motherhood and womanhood had linkages to the African continent. Enslaved women, who were descended from West and Central African ethnic groups, continued to incorporate the cultural practices that their foremothers had taught them about motherhood. These lessons ranged from how to suckle their children to how to wrap them in swaddling cloth while the mothers farmed plots of land. Also, because enslaved people could not legally marry and raise their children in the nuclear family model that was common for white Americans, motherhood took on special significance for black women in ways that marriage did not. Historian Andrew Apter discusses the importance of "blood mothers" in nineteenth-century Yorubaland, southwest Nigeria, and certain parts of Togo, Ghana, and Benin. Apter states, "The model of West African womanhood that took effect in the Americas is associated with the blood of mothers . . . that which gives them the ability to conceive and give birth."[11]

"Blood" served as a metaphor for West African mothers and their descendants who were born in America. It contained both good and bad essences and forged ties among black women that were both secret and sacred. Life and death were contained in the blood, from the release of menstrual blood and blood lost during miscarriages to the symbolic use of blood as a mode for purification.[12] For women who anticipated pregnancy and motherhood because of their significance in their conceptions of womanhood and also their self-worth as fertile women, the intrusion in their lives of white southern men who replaced midwives compromised the deeply personal relationships they had with one another on an ancestral and a cultural level.

Black women viewed themselves as the cultural bearers of West African beliefs about motherhood, but they had to combat negative views that white physicians had about black women's bodies, especially their genitalia. Because doctors believed in the inferiority of women and the double inferiority of black women, they considered natural biological conditions such as menstruation pathological. In the same vein, they also determined that the clitoris was an underdeveloped penis.[13] In an 1810 medical article, Dr. John Archer asserted that the clitorises of little black girls were larger than those of their white peers because they accompanied their enslaved mothers to the fields while they worked. The doctors theorized that because these children sat unattended for long periods, their clitorises developed at a younger age.[14]

In the first half of the nineteenth century, deviancy seemed to define "femaleness." Sadly, this American conception of womanhood, health, and value precluded the importance of the West African "blood mother." It is from these seeds that modern American gynecology germinated into a branch of medicine adorned with both flowers and thorns. Like their peers in eighteenth-century Europe, antebellum-era American doctors who created gynecology began with the belief that "females in general were . . . a sexual subset of their race."[15]

Despite the general belief that black people, especially women, were inferior, the bodies of black women fascinated, as well as repulsed, white southern doctors. American slavery provided abundant opportunities for medical doctors to experiment on and sometimes heal sick bondwomen. Medical doctors happily engaged in experimental medical research that focused on restoring black women's reproductive capabilities, as the following examples illustrate.

In 1835, four doctors, John Bellinger, S. H. Dickson, T. G. Prioleau, T. Ogier, and two medical students, Mr. Tennent and Mr. Frierson, conducted an experimental ovarian surgery on a thirty-five-year-old black slave woman. She was to have an ovarian tumor removed.[16] The woman was the mother of one child, born seven years earlier; she had also suffered a number of miscarriages.

The previous year, the enslaved woman felt a lump on the right side of her abdomen, and since then she had been troubled with pain in her abdominal area. Doctors later diagnosed her as having a tumor. Right before Christmas, her team of doctors performed an ovariotomy to excise her tumor. During the surgery, the doctors realized there was "no opportunity for the safe use of the knife." One of the doctors recorded in his notes that the enslaved patient lost "her self-command, screamed and struggled violently—rendering it no easy task to control her movements and support the viscera."[17] After physically restraining her, the doctors continued the operation. Her recovery was slow, and she later reported that she never again menstruated. Although the procedure had probably made her sterile, thereby decreasing her economic value, her diseased ovary, which was displayed at the Charleston, South Carolina, Medical College's museum, held greater worth for her doctors. This enslaved woman's diseased ovary would be used as a pedagogical tool and a medical curiosity.[18]

In a similar case a decade later, Dr. Raymond Harris, a Georgia physician, was asked by William Patterson, a slave owner in Bryan County, to examine one of his slaves. She had been experiencing uncommon symptoms during her pregnancy. After Harris probed the parturient woman, he found that she had "a large irregular tumor." The woman's menses had ceased for two years, and she had been constipated for months.[19] Harris operated on the thirty-six-year-old mother and determined that she had an ovarian pregnancy. He gave the bondwoman medicine, and her condition improved almost immediately.[20] After some time had elapsed, Harris wrote a medical article. In it he claimed that the enslaved woman's plantation owner and nurse had testified that the bondwoman had successfully regained her menses. Unfortunately, the enslaved woman began to experience the same symptoms she had manifested years before she became Dr. Harris's patient. Harris prescribed a potent dosage of medicine that included "iodide of potassium . . . in 5 gr. doses" to treat the enslaved woman's symptoms. She died shortly thereafter.[21] Upon learning of the woman's death, Harris stated, "Although it was late in the day, and myself much hurried, I requested permission to open the body."[22] He later lamented that he had not saved the enslaved woman's reproductive parts for preservation and study. For early gynecologists like Harris, even postmortem, a bondwoman's "real" value was still measured by her reproductive organs.[23]

Preserving diseased and damaged reproductive parts, performing experimental surgeries, and canvassing slave communities for sick patients helped southern doctors, medical colleges and museums, and their faculty and students advance their medical knowledge quite literally on the broken bodies of black slaves. Prior to the founding of the AMA in 1847, there was no single code of medical ethics. Systems of ethics regarding experimentation on the enslaved were idiosyncratic. In an 1826 issue of the *Philadelphia Journal of Medical and Physical Sciences*, Dr. P. Tidyman advised physicians who treated the enslaved that "it should always be left to the choice of the patient, to go into the hospital or be attended in his house. It [was] the interest and duty of the owner to consult the feelings of the slave."[24] Despite this seemingly polite ritual in southern manners, the practice, even if actually followed, rang hollow for enslaved patients if they did not know what the treatments would do to their bodies. Unfortunately, the ideology of antiblack racism was too ingrained in the culture for southern physicians to heed Dr. Tidyman's admonishments. Even if an enslaved woman stated that she did not want to be operated on, once her owner granted permission to the surgeon to perform surgery, an operation occurred. Medical care of slaves evolved from its beginnings on slave ships to a mostly unregulated behemoth that tended to create "rules" as the field evolved.

Rules and ethical codes were created as new crises cropped up, and some early physicians and surgeons believed that the practice of slave medicine and, more particularly, human experimentation could lead to abuses by medical researchers. Antebellum-era physician William Beaumont created rules for medical research in 1833 "to provide an ethical framework for nontherapeutic trials."[25] Beaumont stipulated the following conditions:

> 1. There must be recognition of an area where experimentation in man is needed . . . 2. Some experimental studies in man are justifiable when the information cannot otherwise be obtained. 3. The investigator must be conscientious and responsible . . . 4. Whenever a human subject is used, a well considered, methodological approach is required so that as much information as possible will be obtained. No random studies are to be made. 5. The voluntary consent of the subject is necessary . . . 6. The experiment is to be discontinued when it cause distress to the subject . . . and 7. The project must be abandoned when the subject becomes dissatisfied.[26]

Although experimentation on enslaved women was extensive, it was almost always therapeutic, since the goal was to enhance reproductive success. Broadly, most doctors who worked on slaves did so to protect, if not increase, the economic interests of slave owners and also to perfect their own skill set as doctors and physicians. The growth of gynecology provided for the maintenance of sound black female reproductive bodies; it also served to perpetuate the institution of slavery. Slavery, medicine, and capitalism were intimate bedfellows.[27]

Bondwomen were aware of their pecuniary worth in slave-trading transactions. They knew that potential slave owners had great interest in whether black women could breed with relative ease and also if they suffered from reproductive ailments that affected their fertility. Thus some enslaved women developed sophisticated measures to demonstrate some agency in their sale on auction blocks. Some would pass themselves off as healthy, even when they knew they had reproductive illnesses and sexually transmitted diseases that affected their fertility. One major advantage for enslaved women who employed this technique might be to escape mean owners, abuse, or simply especially grueling work schedules.

Warranty cases that featured the enslaved often bore these facts out in judicial court proceedings. Slave warranty cases based on redhibition, the legal template from which originated the "lemon laws" allowing legal action against the seller of a defective product, shed light on the various ways in which enslaved women dissembled to fool buyers and new owners.[28] Such a court case in South Carolina offers an example of a black woman's complicity in hiding her illness. In November 1821, a jury deliberated over the case of *Hughes ads. Banks*, in which the new owner of a slave woman, Mr. Banks, charged the previous slave master, Mr. Hughes, with willfully selling him a sick slave. According to court testimony, "Dr. Hammond . . was called in to attend the woman. . . . About seven weeks after the sale, . . [the woman became] excessively ill, and died on the next evening. . . . Hughes acknowledged that the woman had the venerial many years, (12 or 14) before, but had got entirely well; although some of her children had cutaneous eruptions, . . . easily cured."[29] The court found in favor of the defendant. Mr. Hughes received six hundred dollars and court costs for the death of the recently deceased slave woman, who was deemed "defective goods" largely because she had a sexually transmitted disease that affected her health and potential to reproduce.[30] Although the woman is rendered voiceless, it is highly improbable that she did not know that she had a sexually transmitted disease, one that she had for a number of years, as Dr. Hammond, the attending physician, noted. Records do not indicate why she remained silent about her disease, but it is unlikely that the disease manifested no symptoms, especially since her children had developed symptoms.

One year later in 1822, another South Carolina jury deliberated over a similar slave warranty case, *Lightner ads. Martin*, that concerned an enslaved woman who suffered from a sexually transmitted disease. The heart of the case centered on the following assertion: it was "alleged that one of the negroes 'had the venereal disease at the time of sale . . . that this woman had communicated the disease to others of his negroes, by which he had incurred a great loss and expense.' "[31] After the enslaved woman's owner contacted a physician to examine her, the bondwoman was given "a course of medicine" and became healthy. Her owner proceeded to sell her immediately.[32]

The *Lightner ads. Martin* case is distinctive because of the language used to describe the enslaved woman's illness and sexual behavior. Not only was the South Carolinian slave afflicted with a "venereal disease"; according to the language of the case, she was also promiscuous. Her promiscuity was such a threat to the health of the owner's other slaves that she was sold, even after she had been healed. This enslaved black woman's sexual power was perceived to be so potent that she was believed to be capable of creating life and destroying the reproductive value of black life simultaneously. Medical and legal writings such as this one contained explicit language about how devious behavior was mapped onto black women's bodies. Alongside medical journals, judicial cases demonstrate the ongoing struggle of nineteenth-century Americans to define blackness within the realm of reproductive labor and sometimes to establish the sanity of enslaved people. In *Stinson ads. Piper*, the State of South Carolina declared that "a warranty of soundness embraces soundness of mind as well as body." This decision was made because of the questionable "soundness" of a recently purchased slave woman.[33]

The reach of southern medical doctors and slaveholders into black people's lives was so extensive and powerful that they could create illnesses linking the reproductive diseases of black people to their supposed degeneracy as women and mothers. In 1851, Dr. E. M. Pendelton of Hancock, Georgia, presented his research in "The Comparative Fecundity of the Black and White Races." Writing about black women, Pendelton reported, "The blacks are much better breeders than the whites." Yet the doctor offered a confusing reason for why enslaved women have more children: "Our negro females are forever drenching themselves with nostrums, injurious to their health and fatal to their offspring."[34] Despite black women allegedly poisoning themselves and their unborn children with dangerous potions, miraculously, they still managed to have more children than white women in Hancock County. These harmful beliefs represented black people's "soul murder."[35] Formerly enslaved Delia Garlic offered a poignant statement about white people's inhumane treatment of black people. Garlic pronounced, "It's bad to belong to folks dat own you soul and body."[36] Although she was not directly referencing gynecology's development and the research linked to it that understood black women as something other than normal human beings, Garlic's words are applicable to women's medicine.

Despite the ownership of black women's bodies by slave owners, enslaved women did resist the efforts of slave masters to lay claim to their "souls." They did so by sharing long-held folk wisdom and recipes that they used to heal members of slave communities. O. W. Green recalled how his grandmother, a slave nurse, passed along her medical and pharmaceutical knowledge to her family members. Green's grandmother provided thirty-seven years of service as a plantation nurse who doctored "all de young'uns" on the plantation. Green stated, "When old masta wanted grandmother to go on a special case, he would whip her so she wouldn't tell none of his secrets."[37] Although it was Green's grandmother who was giving medical care to patients, her white owner, who was also a doctor, took possession of her knowledge and touted it as his medical "secret" and inflicted corporal punishment on the woman to force her allegiance to him, "body and soul." Yet she defied her master in the privacy of her community and divulged her body of medical and herbal knowledge to her grandson.

Green disclosed his grandmothers "working cures" to his WPA interviewer, in a final act of ancestral defiance. She favored "black snake root, sasparilla, [and] blackberry briar roots" in her roots medicine practice, he told the interviewer.[38]

Although white men and black women were often in conflict over black women's medical treatments, in many instances, white men, both doctors and slave owners, also expected black women to treat expectant mothers and the infirm with the same body of knowledge that these men also derided. Dellie Lewis's grandmother, who was a plantation midwife, provides an example. Lewis revealed a favorite botanically based method that her grandmother employed when working on her parturient patients. The midwife blended a mixture of "cloves and whiskey to ease the pain" of childbirth.[39] Historian Sharla Fett has argued that bondwomen also resisted the wholesale control that slave owners and medical doctors had over their bodies. They "worked cures" noninvasively as they sought to establish a "relational view of healing" for themselves that privileged a more holistic model of healing.[40] Likewise, Julia Brown's narrative corroborates how enslaved women relied on and believed in the healing practices of granny midwives. Brown stated, "We didn't go to no hospitals as they do now. We just had our babies and a granny to catch 'em. We didn't have all the pain-easin' medicines. . . . The granny would put a ax under my mattress once. This was to cut off the after-pains and it sure did, too."[41]

Like enslaved women, most white Americans had little confidence or trust in professional medical care because of its invasive nature. They often became sicker or, even worse, saw their loved ones die under a doctor's care. Such poor outcomes are not surprising, given the haphazard nature of early American medicine. It was not governed by any national organization that created comprehensive regulations and ethical codes for doctors to follow. The AMA was not founded until 1847. One of its initial purposes was to standardize the qualifications of medical doctors. Before the AMA's creation, many men entered the field without formal educational training and little to no practical experience. American medicine harbored as many quacks as reputable health-care providers. For upwardly mobile young white men who bypassed either the ministry or law to practice medicine, their career choice was tantamount, in many regards, to throwing away their future and their respectability.

James Marion Sims's father initially scorned his son's decision to study medicine by stating that the field had "no science to it." To counter this notion, young men like Sims began to merge racial science with medicine as they engaged in experimental surgeries and published their results for the advancement of women's medicine. Dr. Sims's writings exemplify the cognitive dissonance that antebellum American medical men experienced as they wrote about enslaved patients and race. Although these doctors' publications were meant for white audiences only, black people observed and responded to white doctors' participation in reproductive medicine. Most importantly, enslaved women's presence represented more than silent bodies on operating tables even if medical writings attempted to reduce them to one-dimensional objects.

Enslaved women knew that their lives were public and thus they had to protect what little privacy they had, especially with regard to their sicknesses. Thus black women rarely sought the services of white doctors. For those who did, the issue of the woman's consent to surgery was problematic. In the case of Mary, the black surgical patient whose womb Dr. Paul Eve excised, she was asked initially if she wanted to undergo surgery. Eve wrote, "Without persuasion or influence of any kind, she determined promptly and unhesitatingly to submit to the operation."[42] One might ask, however, if Mary, in antebellum-era Georgia, really had the choice of rejecting Dr. Eve's offer. By midcentury, it seems that black women, both free and enslaved, and white male doctors at least participated in a ritual of etiquette that afforded black women the pretense of having a choice about submitting to the proposed surgical procedure.

Within this extremely unequal power system was a parallel black medical practice that enslaved women were sometimes wily enough to engage; many times, however, it failed them. Fortunately, the oral histories of formerly enslaved women and men illuminate a complex medical past that has too often been shrouded in darkness. Their words reveal the myriad practices that black women used when caring for one another and their children. Fannie Moore told how her enslaved grandmother "worked cures" for the entire plantation community.[43] Moore told of how her grandmother used "roots and bark for teas of all kinds" to cure common illnesses. When she treated colicky infants, the elder Moore would "get rats vein and make a syrup and put a little sugar in it and boil it. Den soon as it cold she give it to de baby."[44] The enslaved and their enslavers moved uneasily between two worlds. One world was rooted in the here and now, where formally trained doctors consulted textbooks and articles on the diseases that affected black women and their children, while the other world relied on the folk knowledge and practices of enslaved women. These worldviews often clashed, but there were also synergistic moments.

In one of the earliest scholarly texts on the health of plantation slaves, historian William Dosite Postell wrote, "Uterine troubles were of common occurrence among slave women."[45] A May 1859 judicial warranty case that involved on a Louisiana bondwoman illustrates Dosite Postell's point. In *Gaienne v. Freret*, the plaintiff, Mr. Gaienne, had purchased an allegedly "sound" slave from Mr. Freret on February 3, 1859, in Louisiana. Two weeks after her purchase, the bondwoman alerted her new master that she was, in fact, not sound and suffered from a uterine disease. It was discovered that the woman had an "ulceration of the uterus which she had carefully concealed from her former owner."[46] At Gaienne's request, four physicians examined the enslaved woman and recommended that Gaienne return her to her former owner, Freret, immediately. After the woman was returned to Freret's farm, she underwent another battery of "treatments," this time, in a local hospital.[47] Even though Freret believed that he had hired "skillful physicians" to treat his slave, the woman died soon after her stay in the hospital.[48] We will never know the specific reasons why this bondwoman concealed her uterine disease from her owners; it is conceivable, however, that she might have confided her physical status to one of the black women charged with caring for enslaved women on Freret's plantation. Enslaved women might have been terrified to disclose their health concerns to their owners, not only because of the issues surrounding gender but also because hospitals were often viewed with suspicion and considered sites of death. Historian Elaine Breslaw argues that "doctors carried an aura of death"; when called to assist nurses and midwives, enslaved women were no different in the way they viewed doctors: with great fear.[49]

As both the legal and the medical systems worked out the processes of how black women were to be defined and treated by doctors, jurists, slave owners, and southern society, individual American doctors were adding their perspectives to the discussion, medical case by medical case. Dr. John Archer cautioned physicians, and by extension, slave owners, who treated enslaved women medically to exercise vigilance in their treatments. Archer argued that if white medical men and slave owners did not prioritize the physical care of enslaved women, ultimately, black women would suffer from white men's neglect. He advocated for southern white paternalism without having to invoke the term "father." Thus medical journals could also encourage white men to serve as responsible providers for enslaved women. Archer believed that slave masters should be wedded not to principles of altruism but to practicality. The protection of a healthy black female labor force meant that slavery would not only survive but also thrive.

As the domestic slave trade flourished, enslaved women had to fight continuous intrusions into their reproductive lives. Medicine, especially gynecology, represented one of the largest encroachments black women faced, particularly because of the level of social control that doctors and hospitals exerted over them. Numerous medical journal articles described black failure and inferiority in wide-ranging ways. Doctors discussed the dirty appearance of black female bodies, the inability of black women to cook food properly for their families, and examined so-called black practices such as eating clay or dirt, also termed "cachexia Africana."[50] The reports and articles of these doctors continued to promote a general belief that blackness was unclean and caused disorderliness and that black bodies were vectors of disease. Black people and their "race" represented an oppositional framework for whiteness as represented in American society. Therefore, the ideology of white paternalism aided gynecology's growth by laying claim to black women's reproductive bodies, both metaphorically and literally.

The writing of Kentucky physician John Harrison demonstrates how the presence of white male doctors contributed to furthering ideas about black women's inadequacies as healers. In the opening sentence of Harrison's 1835 article, "Cases in Midwifery," he wrote, "This was a badly managed case at first; for an old ignorant negro midwife had been the first assistant of nature."[51] He was condescending in his description of the "ignorant" black midwife who was involved in an extremely difficult obstetrical case. Five years earlier, Harrison had treated a black patient who was caught in limbo, trapped between life and death. He graphically described a ghastly scene in his article. On December 23, 1830, Harrison "found a black woman . . . lying in bed . . . with part of the forearm and hand of the child hanging out of the vulva." He directed the woman's husband and her elderly enslaved midwife to separate and hold up her legs so that he could deliver the woman's baby.[52] Harrison described the black midwife as inadequately prepared to handle her patient's obstetrical condition, although he had to rely on her assistance during the delivery. Harrison, as a product of the slaveholding South, knew that it was common practice for a slave midwife to deliver enslaved children. The rules created by white supremacy dictated that only a black woman could serve as the "first assistant of nature" in a slave woman's delivery. He was simply finishing a job that the nurse had begun earlier. Harrison's journal article helps to explicate the vulnerability of enslaved women in their roles as patients and nurses.[53]

Black midwives had to serve the interests of slave owners and, later, physicians by acquiescing to the complete authority that these men exercised over them and their charges. As white men became involved in midwifery cases, black midwives began to bear physical witness to the surgical treatment and repair of enslaved women who had given birth. Midwives had always relied on unobtrusive tools to birth babies. When white men integrated obstetrics and gynecology, pregnant enslaved women who experienced difficult birthing processes became disproportionately represented in surgical cases in which doctors used blades and forceps to remove fetuses. Surgeries were quite rare in the first half of the nineteenth century, so it is astounding how many medical journal articles listed enslaved women as surgical patients. Although the archival sources do not provide precise figures for the number of gynecological surgeries performed during the nineteenth century, one can assume that these sorts of operations occurred with more frequency than has been reported.

Statistics compiled from two leading medical and surgical journals of the era, the *American Journal of Medical Sciences* (AJMS) and the *Boston Medical and Surgical Journal* (BMSJ), over a twenty-year period (1830–50) reveal that enslaved women underwent a number of intrusive gynecological operations performed by doctors.[54] The numbers do not determine if enslaved women were operated on more often than white women in the South, but had they been free, the percentages of surgeries this population experienced would have been smaller. The surgeries that were published about enslaved women featured a large number of sexual procedures. During the twenty-year span under consideration, AJMS published only two case narratives provided by physicians on the experimental nature of their surgeries and/or autopsies, both in 1850. The first case involved an operation on the corpse of a recently deceased enslaved woman; the second case recorded the medical findings following the complete removal of a deceased slave's uterus. Early gynecological surgeries reported in the journal in 1830, 1835, 1840, and 1845 did not contain citations referencing experimental sexual surgeries performed on enslaved women. After James Marion Sims's pioneering 1852 article on vesico-vaginal fistulae appeared in the AJMS, the number of medical articles on sexual surgeries on all women published by the journal increased by more than 100 percent.

Between 1830 and 1850, only four articles explicitly addressing black women's reproductive health issues appeared in the *Boston Medical and Surgical Journal*.[55] Two of the articles appeared in 1835, in the February and July issues. The first piece detailed the dissection of a black woman's reproductive organs during an autopsy, and the second article described a seemingly unbelievable medical feat: a fourteen-year old enslaved Jamaican teenaged girl performed a cesarean section on herself. Five years later, in the April 15, 1840, issue of the BMSJ, John Peter Mettauer wrote the editorial staff about his "pioneering" and successful surgery to repair the common nineteenth-century "women's ailment" vesico-vaginal fistula. Mettauer reported that his patient, a slave, had recuperated and remained healthy during the two years that had elapsed since he performed the experimental surgery. Mettauer also asked the journal's editors if they could check their records to make sure he would be known as the first physician-surgeon in the country to successfully perform the operation. Last, in October 1845, an autopsy was performed on an enslaved woman's corpse to view her damaged reproductive organs.

One medical case reported by Dr. John Bellinger, in the *Southern Journal of Medicine and Pharmacy*, detailed the surgery he had performed on an unidentified enslaved woman. In the late eighteenth century, an elderly African-born woman was brought to the doctor because of her extreme vaginal pain.[56] After he performed an initial vaginal examination, Bellinger determined that her symptoms derived from the "very small opening" in her vagina. The bondwoman intimated that she had lived with the pain her entire life; she was then ninety years old. Bellinger found that her vagina was completely obliterated, and as a result, the woman had trouble urinating. Probably feigning ignorance, the woman responded to the doctor's probing questions about how she came to be in her condition with an answer that pointed to her having "no history of the affair at all."[57] She may have been playing "hush mout," a feature of the culture of dissemblance in which enslaved women used silence for their survival and protection within slave communities. The physician performed regular procedures, for nearly ten years, to correct her condition and lessen the patient's physical pain. After she reached nearly one hundred years old, she endured a number of operations to remove "small urinary concretions or calculi" from her vaginal area.[58]

Clearly, this elderly enslaved woman had no real economic value for her owner; she was past the age of fecundity and could not reproduce. Dr. Bellinger, however, had full access to the woman's body for nearly a decade. Although he asserted that she had confided in him that her pain was relieved after undergoing ten years' worth of vaginal examinations and operations, Bellinger continued to treat his enslaved patient so that he could publish an article in one of the country's leading medical journals, the *Southern Journal of Medicine and Pharmacy*.[59] Medical doctors published articles for various reasons, education, self-promotion, and to build a body of work that could advance a burgeoning field, and Bellinger's motives were likely no different.

The enslaved woman on whom Bellinger conducted his research occupied a far different place in antebellum society. Elderly black women were deemed worthless in a society that prized black females for their presumed hypersexuality and reproductive abilities. A review of an appraisement roster compiled by South Carolina physician and slave owner James Spann in 1838 elucidates how enslaved women were assessed financially, especially elderly ones. For example, "1 Negro Woman Called Rose" was worth one dollar, an indication that she was probably aged or infertile.[60] Rose was priced less than James Spann's "Two Tubs and 1 Churn." According to the dictates of antebellum white southern society, any elderly, barren, or ailing female slave represented an economic loss within the slave market economy.[61] In the medical case of Dr. Bellinger's patient, however, her damaged vagina was worthwhile because it helped to advance the growing body of knowledge within gynecology.

Recalling the 1824 case of the pregnant teenage rape victim who was treated by Dr. John Harrison also helps us grasp how important the production and publication of obstetrical and gynecological knowledge was for American physicians. A.P. was a fifteen-year-old enslaved girl owned by a Louisville, Kentucky, master; she had become pregnant after being raped by a local white man. Her pregnancy was difficult, and the physical challenges lasted through her delivery, when she suffered painful contractions.[62] Harrison bled A.P. for a length of time until she convulsed and fainted. Further complicating her delivery was the fact that the teenage slave was carrying twins. The doctor decided "nothing but delivery could save the patient," and he commenced with the immediate removal of her twins.[63] Although Harrison provided obstetrical care when A.P.'s enslaved midwife believed the girl would die, he published an article that presented him as an expert in midwifery, although he unknowingly compromised her health with his reliance on bloodletting.

A.P.'s case is a harrowing one because of the results of her rape, birthing mulatto twins while undergoing a torturous birthing process. Even when black women were forced into sexual relationships with black men, their decisions to identify their abusers are powerful reminders of how slavery and reproduction intersected. Unknown numbers of enslaved women became pregnant from these violent encounters, and for women like A.P.'s midwife and Louisa Everett, their disclosures of sexual abuse were strong counternarratives to black women's supposed lasciviousness.

Everett, who was formerly owned by Jim McClain of Norfolk, Virginia, provided a testimony of her experience as a victim of sexual abuse to her WPA interviewer. Mrs. Everett's candor was unusual because many black women dissembled about their sexual lives and experiences under southern slavery. Everett stated in explicit detail how her former owner forced his slaves to perform in orgies for him and his friends. She recalled,

> Marse Jim called me and Sam ter him and ordered Sam to pull off his shirt—that was all the McClain niggers wore—and he said to me: Nor, "do you think you can stand this big nigger?" He had that old bull whip flung acrost his shoulder, and Lawd, that man could hit so hard! . . . "Yassur, I guess so," . . . Well he told us what we must git busy and do in his presence, and we had to do it. After that we were considered man and wife. Me and Sam was a healthy pair and had fine, big babies, so I never had another man forced on me, thank God. Sam was kind to me and I learnt to love him.[64]

The couple's rape, meant to "breed slave children" and sexually titillate their master and his friends, opens a lens on the sexual abuse sustained by enslaved women and, in this case, enslaved men. Within the American landscape of slavery, Mrs. Everett's narrative reveals the traumatic aftereffects of sexual abuse and exploitation that enslaved women had to contend with, including depression, pregnancy, and in some cases infectious diseases that were venereal in origin. Despite the horrifying experiences that Everett endured, she was able to eventually create a loving relationship with her husband, Sam, and their children.

The joyful way that she spoke of her family offers testimony to the resiliency that enslaved women were forced to develop as a counter to slavery's dehumanization of black and white people. The beliefs that slave owners held about black women's inability to distinguish between corporeal pleasure and pain is echoed in Everett's account. Slave women's words intimate that their lives should not be encapsulated into neat and unsatisfactory binary categories of either victim or resistor. One should keep in mind David Morris's assertion that "pain . . . is always more than a matter of nerves and neurotransmitters" when attempting to understand the multidimensionality of black women's medical and sexual lives.[65]

The rampant sexual abuse of enslaved women by white men was common knowledge throughout southern society, but although the practice was scorned, little was done to curb it. One of the ways in which enslaved women and their black male partners attempted to restore love and humanity in their lives and relationship was to engage in mutually satisfying sexual partnerships with each other and to plan their pregnancies. Legal scholar Dorothy Roberts found that enslaved women tended to "became pregnant during the months of November, December, and January when labor requirements were reduced owing to completion of the harvest and to harsh weather."[66] In a random sampling of over one hundred slave interviews, 26.73 percent of interviewees are registered by their birth month and year.[67] Concurrent with these findings, the majority of births listed within the data set occurred during the beginning of agricultural crop seasons; 14.81 percent of respondents cited March, May, September, and November as their birth months.[68] This sample suggests that enslaved women quite possibly exercised some control over their conceptions. Lapses in their work schedules, especially during noncrop seasons, allowed bondwomen to manage when they would conceive.[69]

Enslaved women understood that the contours of enslavement did not grant them full freedom to prevent physicians from performing risky medical procedures on them or administering drugs that often proved fatal during pregnancy and the postnatal period. But for bondwomen, planned pregnancies implied a sense of liberation because they could determine the pre- and postnatal care that they would receive from black midwives. An 1846 medical journal article, authored by physician P. C. Gaillard, detailed that he visited an unidentified enslaved woman after she reported to her master that her newborn was severely ill. The slave mother confided to Gaillard that her "child was as carefully attended from its birth as possible" because the infant signified the slave woman's final "planned pregnancy."[70] She had given birth eleven years earlier, and at forty years old, she had decided that this pregnancy would be her final one. Her admission to Gaillard that she had planned her last pregnancy indicates that some enslaved women did exercise control over their reproduction. Also she defended herself against the doctor's accusation that she had killed her baby shortly after its birth. As much as doctors prized black women for their fecundity, they also blamed them when babies developed sicknesses and, in cases such as this one, died.

Even when slave sources do not allow for an examination or an easy interpretation of whether enslaved women planned pregnancies, it is apparent that pregnancy and motherhood transformed how slave owners and doctors treated black women. In some instances, women who had given birth were selected to enter into midwifery and nursing, as they did on the Glover family plantations, owned by siblings Joseph and Edward, in Colleton County, South Carolina. Statistics culled from the Glover family records show how black women were labeled according to their occupations and economic value. The Glover brothers owned three plantations, Mount Pleasant, Richfield, and Swamp. The two of them also owned over 150 enslaved men and women. From 1847 through 1850, the increase in the slave populations on the three plantations was relatively slow but steady. Most Glover slave births occurred in the fall between August and September. Black women conceived on the Glover plantations during winter months, when the pace of agricultural labor had decreased significantly.

Joseph Glover's Richfield Plantation never housed more than seventy-two slaves, and in four years the number of slaves increased only 5.18 percent. Edward Glover owned sixty-four slaves; the slave population on his plantation grew by an average of 5.43 percent. Birthrates ranged from four births in a given year to as low as two births. Only one instance of an infant's death appears in the record, in 1849. The two brothers kept meticulous census accounts of their slaves, and they recorded each slave birth. Although slave births were recorded, the Glovers did not identify the parents of the following slave children who were born during the four-year period: Silvy, Allen, Justice, Lissett, Millan, Minges, Will, Stephan, Mary, Richard, Toby, Nancy, Patty, Hector, Hetty, Peggy, Mary, Cresky (died), Elsey, Miley, Primus, Adam, Lissy, Ansell, Sara, Hector, and Tenah. It is worth noting that some children did share the same names as adult slaves on the plantation.[71]

What is striking about the records the Glovers left is how regularly they used the services of enslaved women on their plantations as nurses and assistant nurses. These women, listed as "Old Lizzett, Old Peg, Maria, Prissy, Hagar, and Phoebe," served the needs of members of their large plantations while also coping with their own gynecological conditions. Lizzett and Peg labored into their senior years as nurses while "working cures" to heal sick members of their plantation communities. Within the time span covered in this study, this core group of enslaved women labored as nurses for fifteen years, from 1844 through 1859, despite being diagnosed by their owners as "infirmed" because of a "falling of the wombs."[72] (Table 2.1 lists the Glover slaves.)

TABLE 2.1 Health and Sale Statuses of Richland and Mount Pleasant Plantation Slaves

Casebook entry date	Name*	Job	Condition	Sale status
January 18,1844	Lizzett (J)	No Report	"Infirm"	same
November 15, 1846	Phoebe (J)	½ hand	"Diseased"	same
November 15, 1846	Peg (J)	½ hand	"Falling of the Womb"	same
November 15, 1846	Melia (J)	½ hand	"Falling of the Womb"	same
November 15, 1846	Scilia (E)	½ hand	"Falling of the Womb"	same
November 20, 1847	Lissett (J)	½ hand	"Infirm"	same
November 20, 1847	Phoebe (J)	½ hand	No Report	No Report
November 20, 1847	Peg (J)	½ hand	"Diseased"	same
November 20, 1847	Melia (J)	½ hand	"Diseased"	same
November 20, 1847	Scilla (E)	½ hand	"Diseased"	same
November 20, 1847	Maria (E)	Nurse	N/A	same
November 1848	Lissett (J)	½ hand	"Infirm"	same
November 1848	Phoebe (J)	½ hand	"Diseased"	same
November 1848	Peg (J)	½ hand	"Diseased"	same
November 1848	Melia (J)	½ hand	"Diseased"	same
November 1848	Scilla (E)	½ hand	"Diseased"	same
November 1848	O Caty (E)	½ hand	"Infirm"	same
November 1848	Maria (E)	Nurse	N/A	same
January 25, 1851	O Caty (E)	No report	"Infirm"	same
January 25, 1851	Maria (E)	Nurse	N/A	same
January 25, 1851	Phoebe (J)	½ hand	"Falling of the Womb"	same
January 28, 1851	Melia (E)	½ hand	"Falling of the Womb"	Sold for $263
November 22, 1851	Old Peg (E)	Nurse	No report	Bought by E. Glover
January 5, 1852	Phoebe (J)	½ hand	"Falling of the Womb"	same
January 25, 1853	Phoebe (J)	½ hand	"Falling of the Womb"	same
January 28, 1853	Peg (J)	½ hand	"Falling of the Womb"	same
January 28, 1853	Prissy (J)	Asst. nurse	No report	Appears sold to J. Glover
January 28, 1853	O'Peg (J)	Nurse	No report	same
January 28, 1853	Maria (E)	Nurse	N/A	same
January 12, 1854	Maria (E)	Nurse	N/A	same
January 13, 1854	O Lizzett (J)	Nurse	No report	No report except now called "old"

TABLE 2.1 (continued)

Casebook entry date	Name*	Job	Condition	Sale status
January 13, 1854	Phoebe (J)	Nurse	No report	Repaired
January 13, 1854	Prissy (J)	Asst. nurse	No report	same
January 10, 1855	O Lizzett (J)	Nurse	No report	same
January 10, 1855	Phoebe (J)	Nurse	No report	same
January 10, 1855	Prissy (J)	Asst. nurse	No report	same
January 1, 1856	O Lizzett (J)	Nurse	"Very Old"	same
January 1, 1856	Phoebe (J)	Nurse	No report	same
January 1, 1856	Prissy (J)	Asst. nurse	No report	same
January 11, 1856	Maria (E)	Nurse	N/A	same
January 11, 1856	Hagar (E)	Asst. nurse at the Swamp (another plantation)	N/A	same
January 6, 1857	O Lizzett (J)	Nurse	"Very Old"	same
January 6, 1857	Phoebe (J)	Nurse	No report	same
January 6, 1857	Prissy (J)	Asst. nurse	No report	same
January 1, 1858	O Lizzett (J)	No job reported	"Very Old"	same
January 1, 1858	Phoebe (J)	Nurse	No report	same
January 1, 1858	Prissy (J)	Asst. nurse	No report	same
January 1, 1859	O Lizzett (J)	No job	No report	same
January 1, 1859	Phoebe (J)	Nurse	No report	same
January 1, 1859	Prissy (J)	Nurse	No report	same
January 1, 1859	Orinter (E)	¼ hand	"very old infirm"	same
January 1, 1859	Maria (E)	Nurse	N/A	same

Source: Glover Family Papers.

*The initials in parentheses indicate whether the slave belonged to John (J) or Edward (E) Glover.

Phoebe's transition from patient to nurse is interesting because of how she was described and listed by her owners. She was first described by the generic term "diseased." A few years later, Phoebe's uterus prolapsed. By 1859, she was described by the work she performed on the plantation, "nurse." On the Glover plantations, Phoebe shared similar life patterns with many of the women assigned to work as plantation nurses. They first toiled as field hands. After experiencing illness, usually a gynecological one, these bondwomen became plantation nurses. Most slaves were agricultural laborers, so the fact that the Glovers' owned so many women who were nurses illustrates how regularly the enslaved on their three plantations became ill.

Figures 2.1–3 are records from the Glover family plantation books showing how sick bondwomen transitioned into nursing. Old Lizzett, who is listed as number 13 in the ledger, had an illness in January 1851 that reduced her value so greatly that in the section under "hands" her box was left blank (see fig. 2.1). Old Lizzett's age along with her illness probably affected her ability to perform work like the other Glover slave hands. Phoebe, who is listed as number 22 in the ledger book, had a fallen womb. Her gynecological condition had her valued at ½ hand status, which indicates that her labor output was reduced by half because of her condition. By the next year, Old Lizzett was back to nursing, and so was Phoebe. Melia, another slave on one of the Glover plantations, was sold in 1851, along with eighteen others, for $263. She was the only enslaved woman whose entry on the list included a reason for her being sold, "falling of womb" (see fig. 2.3)

The surviving records do not indicate how these women gained their medical training and expertise. However, many enslaved women provided medical care to one another and their community members, so it is quite possible that older midwives might have chosen younger women whom they were close to, had shared medical experiences with, or were related to. Importantly, just as enslaved women in Colleton County, South Carolina, worked as midwives and nurses in 1859, formal gynecology pioneered by white men was also moving ahead.

Enslaved nurses such as Old Lizzett, Old Peg, and Phoebe also trained younger enslaved women like Prissy in the healing arts. Table 2.1 provides information on what happened to sick women on the Glover plantations as slaves were transitioned from patients in their "sick beds" to plantation nurses as they worked in the "sick house." Those who were deemed "inferior," like Melia, a half-hand field worker, were sold (see Table 2.1, casebook entry for Jan. 28, 1851).[73] Melia, who was owned by Edward Glover, fetched a low price of only $263. In fact, the Glover brothers kept a list of "worthless" slaves and titled the records of these people "List of Inferior Negroes."[74] Many of the women were indexed as having reproductive ailments like Melia. As plantation owners rid themselves of undesirable and "inferior" slaves, those who provided value were used until they could no longer be exploited. The slave nurses, like Old Peg and Phoebe, were on call day and night to care for members of their plantation communities and sometimes local townsfolk who fell ill. South Carolinian Harry McMillan recalled that women "in the family way" on his plantation worked with the same physical intensity as male slaves in the fields. When a parturient enslaved woman "was taken in labor in the field some of her sisters would help her home." McMillan stated that "an old midwife . . . attended them."[75]

A list of the Negroes received by Jos Glov[er]
the 25th of January 1851 —

No	Names	Hands	Remarks
1	Lucy	1	
2	Hannah	1	
3	Chloe	c	Born Feb 9th 1844 ⎫ Sold Jan 2
4	Mingo	c	Born in 1846 ⎪
5	Patty	c	Born in 1849 ⎭
6	Hector	1	
7	Hannah	1	
8	Freeman		Put to carpenter trade 13th of Ja
9	Jenah	c	
10	Liddy	c	Born in 1845
11	Silvey	c	Born July 1847
12	Hector	c	Born 28th of Nov 1849
13	Old Lizzett		In prime
14	Silvey	1	
15	Jinney	c	
16	Lavinia	c	
17	Hannah	c	
18	Hetty	c	Born in 1849
19	Primus	c	Born 2nd of June 1850
20	Edward	1	
21	Dandy	1	
22	Phebe	½	Falling of the womb
23	Eliza	½	
24	Joe	c	
25	Flora	c	Born in 1845
26	Munjer	c	Born in 1848
27	Old Rachel		Poultry minder —

FIGURE 2.1 List of slaves owned by Joseph Glover, 1851.

Glover Family Papers, South Caroliniana Library,
University of South Carolina.

A List of my Negroes on Mt Pleasant Jan 1st 1856

No	Names	Hands	Allowance	Remarks	6th	Clothing Rets
1	Sam		1	Driver	9	
2	Nelly	1	1		6	
3	Dick	1	1		6	
4	Sue	1	1		6	
5	Stephen		4		4	B
6	Nannie		4		3	B
7	Amelia	1	1		6	
8	Lucky		4	died Oct 9th 1856	3	B
9	Hector		1	Stock minder	6	
10	Hannah	1	1		6	
11	Freeman		1	Carpenter	6	
12	Tenah	1/4	6		6	B
13	Liddy		4		4	B
14	Silvey		4		3	B
15	Hector		4		3	B
16	Kate		4		3	B
17	Rinchy		4	Born Sept 21st 1855	3	B
18	Lizzie		1	Nurse, very old	6	
19	Silvey	1	1		6	
20	Jinnie	1/2	1		6	
21	Lavinia		4		4	B
22	Hannah		4		3	B
23	Hetty		4		3	B
24	Edward	1	1		6	
25	Phoebe		1	Nurse	9	
26	Eliza			House Servant	6	
27	Joe		6	Poultry minder	5	B

FIGURE 2.2. List of slaves owned by Joseph Glover,
along with their occupations, 1851.

Glover Family Papers, South Caroliniana Library,
University of South Carolina.

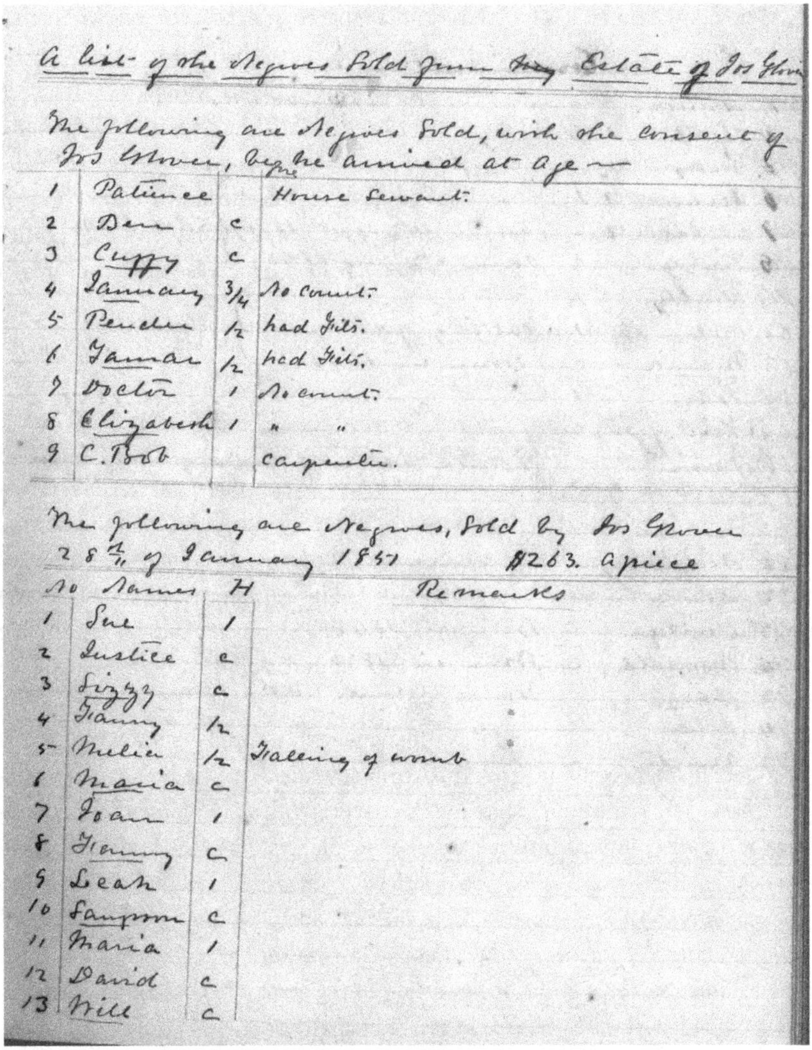

A list of the Negroes Sold from Estate of Jos Glover

The following are Negroes Sold, with the consent of Jos Glover, before he arrived at age —

1	Patience		House servant.
2	Ben	c	
3	Cuffy	c	
4	January	3/4	No count.
5	Pender	1/2	had fits.
6	Tamar	1/2	had fits.
7	Doctor	1	No count.
8	Elizabeth	1	" "
9	C. Bob		carpenter.

The following are Negroes, Sold by Jos Glover 28th of January 1851 $263. apiece

No	Names	H	Remarks
1	Sue	1	
2	Justice	c	
3	Lizzy	c	
4	Fanny	1/2	
5	Melia	1/2	Falling of womb
6	Maria	c	
7	Joan	1	
8	Fanny	c	
9	Leah	1	
10	Sampson	c	
11	Maria	1	
12	David	c	
13	Will	c	

FIGURE 2.3. List of slaves sold by Joseph Glover, 1851.
Melia was sold because of her fallen womb.

Glover Family Papers, South Caroliniana Library,
University of South Carolina.

Two decades later, a Mississippi planter shared with other slave owners that he sent his sick "negroes" to his "large and comfortable" slave hospital to be taken care of by "a very experienced and careful negro woman."[76] There is little doubt that this slave owner, who bragged that he had "not lost a hand since the summer of 1845 (except one . . . killed by accident)," treasured the expertise of his very capable and skilled slave nurse. The master added that his "physician's bill averaged fifty dollars a year."[77] Maintaining enslaved bodies and extending the lives of slaves yielded a palpable increase in the net worth of slave owners.

In southern states, slave owners knew full well the "added value of females due to their ability to generate capital gains."[78] Birthing slaves depended on two factors: an increase in birthrates among enslaved women and the maintenance of bondwomen's reproductive health. Table 2.2 compares the prices of both male and female slaves in six southern states over a one-year period, 1859–60. The slaves included in this comparison lived in Virginia, South Carolina, Georgia, Alabama, Mississippi, and Texas. Of the indexed females whose ages were listed, all but one were presumably of childbearing age. The table shows that in Georgia, South Carolina, and Texas, slave women could be as valuable as highly prized male slaves. In one of the South Carolina cases, a young slave girl was valued at $1,705.

WPA slave narratives and slave management journals contain numerous accounts linking economic growth, pregnancy rates, and medicine. It is incorrect, however, to attribute white men's concern with slave women's reproductive and gynecological health care to benevolence. The solicitude that slave owners exhibited concerning the health of black women's wombs was tied to the bankability of the women's reproductive capability, and not their owners' magnanimity. The action of Mr. James Conway, a Danville, Virginia, slave owner illustrates this point. Responding to the urgent exhortations of one of his pregnant slaves, a thirty-five-year-old married mother, Conway attempted to heal her himself. Because she had given birth previously, Conway must have valued her ability to reproduce. He first bled the sick bondwoman, gave her a laxative, and then administered laudanum "to prevent abortion."[79]

The women who performed the essential duties of birthing babies and saving valuable slave lives were also skilled laborers. Many of their illnesses stemmed from having to perform both reproductive and manual labor. An anonymous overseer from South Carolina wrote in an 1828 slave management manual about the ineffectiveness of physicians and surgeons and recommended training slave women to provide health care when possible. He opined, "An intelligent woman will in a short time learn the use of medicine."[80] As noted earlier, an examination of the varied agricultural labor and health care ser-

TABLE 2.2 Prices of Male and Female Slaves, 1859 and 1860

State and year	Age	Description	Price of male slave	Price of female slave
Alabama, 1859	19		$1,635	
Georgia, 1859		Cotton hand, house servant		$1,250
South Carolina, 1859		Field hand	$1,555	
Texas, 1859	17, 14		$1,527	$1,403
Alabama, 1860	18, 18, 18			$1,193
Georgia, 1860	21	Best field hand	$1,900	
Georgia, 1860	17	With nine-month-old infant		$2,150
Georgia, 1860		Prime, young	$1,300	
Mississippi, 1860		No. 1 field hand	$1,625*	$1,450*
South Carolina, 1860		Prime	$1,325	
South Carolina, 1860		Wench		$1,283
South Carolina, 1860		Girl		$1,705
Texas, 1860	21, 15		$2,015	$1,635
Virginia, 1860	17–20	Best	$1,350–$1,425*	$1,275–$1,325*

Source: Woodman, *Slavery and the Southern Economy*, 89.

*Based on average price listing.

vices that the Glovers' bondwomen performed reveals some interesting data. Enslaved women who worked on the Glover plantations as nurses typically suffered from reproductive conditions prior to becoming nurses and midwives. On the Glovers' plantations, at least two or three younger slave women served as apprentices to plantation nurses. These records reveal that owners valued women who provided this kind of labor and allowed for their training over the years. Further, when historians reassess which slaves were considered skilled laborers, plantation nurses and midwives must be included in their accounting.

Aunt Philis, an elderly slave who lived on the Pope Plantation near Port Royal, South Carolina, shared her thoughts about black women's health care on her plantation. She was convinced that slave masters' demands on pregnant slave women had a negative impact on fetal development and rendered the women unable to produce milk for their infants. Aunt Philis stated, "Dey used to make we work, work, work, so poor moder hab nuffin to gib her child—child starve 'fore it born—dat's what make 'em lean, like buzzard."[81]

Adeline Johnson, who was enslaved in Winnsboro, South Carolina, reported that her doctor, Henry Gibson, worked pregnant enslaved women in the fields until they were near delivery. Johnson declared, "Yes, women in family way worked up to near the time, but guess Dr. Gibson knowed his business. Just before the time, they was took out and put in the carding and spinning rooms."[82]

On Hopedale Plantation, in the Richland district of South Carolina, women performed the same labor as male field hands, picking and chopping cotton. During a three-month period, bondwomen surpassed their male cohorts in terms of the individual amounts of cotton picked on three separate occasions, though they represented on average only 37.06 percent of the total field-hand population on the Hopedale Plantation. Table 2.3 provides a statistical breakdown of the amount of work performed by a typical Hopedale Plantation slave field hand. The statistics do not reveal whether the women working in the cotton fields were pregnant, but it can be assumed that some probably were.

Bondwomen Jenny and Mary, who were field hands on this plantation, routinely outperformed their male counterparts, sometimes picking upward of 781 pounds. If these women were pregnant, the sheer amount of physical labor they performed hoeing, picking, and chopping cotton certainly had the potential to impact negatively their reproductive health and pregnancies. Even while in the fields, many enslaved women were dressed improperly in clothes that provided little protection against bug bites, the heat, and the sharp features of the mature cotton plant. Delia Garlic remarked, "I never had a undershirt until just before my first child was borned. I never had nothin' but a shimmy and a slip for a dress."[83]

Enslaved men also observed the ways that black women suffered from white intrusion and exploitation and how the women supported those among them who were "in the family way." In an interview years after his enslavement, Sam Polite recalled, "She have midwife for nine day and sometime don't have to work for month when baby born."[84] His comments about the medical treatment and recovery of pregnant bondwomen on his former plantation shed light on enslaved black women's practice of seeking privacy within homosocial spaces. Yet the privacy that enslaved women desired during childbirth was depended on their white owners' allowance. For example, on July 13, 1862, an Alabama physician recorded his frustrations about a black midwife's alleged misdiagnosis of an enslaved woman's contractions: "This case had been seen two or three times in the last month by a midwife fearing that she would not do well. They sent for me at which time labor was completed without any trouble."[85] Clearly the pregnant woman was in the throes of such a painful delivery that her midwife requested the doctor's services, a relatively rare occurrence. Yet the doctor dismissed the pregnant bondwoman's pain as stemming from constipation. He could not imagine that the expectant woman might have been experiencing early and false labor pains, which is a common occurrence.

TABLE 2.3 Comparison of Quantity of Cotton Picked per Week according to Slave's Gender

Date	Percentage of hands who were female	Percentage of hands who were male	Total pounds of cotton picked by women (and percentage of total picked)	Total pounds of cotton picked by men (and percentage of total picked)	Pounds picked per woman	Pounds picked per man
August 25, 1852	37 percent	63 percent	4,359 (40.78 percent)	6,331 (59.22 percent)	335.30	287.70
September 2, 1852	37 percent	63 percent	4,435 (39.41 percent)	6,818 (60.59 percent)	341.15	309.90
October 1852	41.2 percent	58.8 percent	4,251 (40.7 percent)	6,191 (59.3 percent)	303.64	309.55
October 1852	34.4 percent	65.6 percent	4,175 (36.51 percent)	7,262 (63.49 percent)	379.55	345.81
October 1852	36.4 percent	63.6 percent	4,630 (35.1 percent)	8,809 (64.9 percent)	396.92	419.48
October 1852	36.4 percent	63.6 percent	5,980 (40.87 percent)	8,651 (59.13 percent)	498.33	411.95

Source: Record and Account Book, 1852–1858, James Davis Trezevant Papers.

The work week for men and women who picked cotton ranged from Monday through Saturday on the Hopedale Plantation. Sunday was the only day that masters did not force their slaves to pick the crop.

The careful management of reproduction by the antebellum slavocracy proved financially lucrative. Bondwomen were acutely aware of their roles in this industry and abetted it by acting as mediators of their own bodies with one another, their lovers, plantation nurses, mistresses, and owners. Sometimes, as Adele Frost recounted, they worked alongside their mistresses. On Adele's Parker's Ferry Plantation, South Carolina, they did not have a doctor. Her "missus and one of the slaves would attend to the sick."[86]

Reproductive medicine proved to be capacious enough to include almost every member of the slave community except black men, who were neither consulted nor considered, at least in medical journal articles, about the medical lives of black enslaved women. An important aspect of bearing children for enslaved women derived from the complex West African meanings of womanhood and motherhood that were attached to their intimate and loving relationships with black men. Marriah Hines relished the fact that her master wed her luckily "to one of the best colored men in the world."[87] She boasted to her interviewer that she had "five chullun by him."[88]

In spite of the joy some enslaved women experienced by having children, others could only lament the brutal and painful impact of slavery on their lives. Mary Reynolds very candidly stated, "Slavery was the worst days was ever seed in the world. They was things past tellin'. . . . I seed worse than what happened to me."[89] Reynolds's secrecy about "things past tellin'" demonstrates how dissemblance aided black women in emotionally reckoning with a system that could very well affect their sanity.

Enslaved women's determined insistence on reproductive autonomy and parental authority pushed forth a slave liberation doctrine that stressed their humanness, strength, resiliency, and intelligence. Despite the boundaries of status and ownership, many bondwomen continued to express feelings of overwhelming joy about motherhood as they sought to plan families. With a combination of thought, planning, and cunningness, female slaves challenged and questioned the notion of slaves as merely movable property, with no power over their reproductive lives. Instead, enslaved women risked the breakup of their families and even the threat of violence in order to birth children on their terms. All the while, enslaved women continued to negotiate their places within this new branch of medicine.

Some enslaved women were defiant in their choice to doctor other bondwomen, like Rena Clark, a slave nurse. The Lafayette County, Mississippi, slave proved far more essential to her owner as a plantation midwife and nurse than his agricultural workers because the specialized labor she provided earned especially high profits. Further, Clark noted that her mistress, Rebecca Pegues, taught her to read when she was twelve years old, and by fifteen years of age,

Rena had became the plantation's midwife, no small feat. After some time, Nick Pegues allowed her to service the local white community. Proud of her work doctoring women, Clark identified herself as an "herb doctor" who could cure almost any woman's ailment. She declared defiantly that she did not "fool wid doctoring no mens," explaining, "I don't know nothin' about their ailments. It always looked like dey could take care of deyselves anyhow. I just doctors women troubles."[90] Unabashedly proud of her specialized work in women's medicine, as a "mother of gynecology," Clark made contributions that paved the way for later black women thinkers and writers like novelist Alice Walker, who coined the word "womanist," the racially and gender-rooted term to describe black feminist concerns.[91] Rena Clark's work stemmed from the dismal realities that bondwomen faced within enslavement. She invoked a deep connection to West African healing practices by using the term "herb doctor" instead of "midwife" to describe herself. By doing so, she revealed how the secular and the sacred interacted in the ways that black women healers viewed themselves.[92]

As much as they could, enslaved black women planned and aborted pregnancies, engaged in sexual relationships with men they chose to love, and passed on medicinal knowledge to their loved ones despite the threat of physical punishment and retaliation by doctors and slave masters. In the examples provided earlier, enslaved midwives reported black women's rapes and tried to protect their reputations and the lives of black mothers and children by requesting the services of white doctors whom they knew their owners respected; during slow periods in their work schedules, they conceived children with black men they loved. When ill, enslaved women brought their weakened bodies and damaged psyches with them to doctor's offices; they presented their fragility as a counter to the damaging ideologies and narratives that "othered" their supposedly stronger black bodies.[93]

Formal institutions of healing such as medical colleges and hospitals, whose doctors increasingly viewed the enslaved as "clinical matter," were the domains of white men; yet enslaved women exercised some agency, as best they could, in their sick houses because white doctors were often absent in these spaces. Black women also knew that sick houses provided relief from agricultural labor and unceasing domestic duties because in them they could recuperate without performing grueling labor. They possessed a sophisticated understanding of uncertain risks, exploitation, and the sometimes-brutal medical treatments they endured by doctors.

As gynecology developed, the relationships that enslaved women had with their owners and doctors served as one of the blueprints for the medical field. A major part of enslaved women's discontent over how their bodies were treated in medicine originated in the sexual relations between these women and white men. The records of the sexual abuse of black women are voluminous, and sources evidence how some bondwomen suffered physically from many of these brutal sexual encounters with white men (and sometimes fellow enslaved men). Therefore, one can infer that once white southern men entered the medical field and began working on black women's bodies, enslaved women were confronted with having to work through a plethora of emotional responses such as hesitancy, resistance, despair, and fear. The contested relations around sex and black women, gynecology's birth, and slavery's growth are inextricably entwined with the emergence of women's professional medicine in the antebellum era.

CHAPTER THREE

CONTESTED RELATIONS

Slavery, Sex, and Medicine

> Before striking me, master questioned me about the
> girl. . . . I only knew that she had been with child, and that
> now she was not, but I did not tell them even of that.
>
> —Mrs. John Little, recounting her silence about a bondwoman's abortion

IN AUGUST 1831, A YOUNG ENSLAVED GIRL, OWNED BY MRS. LEGAY OF
Christ Church Parish, South Carolina, underwent one of the most traumatic experiences imaginable: an enslaved man brutally raped and sodomized
her. The slave girl's physical damage was so extensive that she was unable to
urinate for a week after her rape, her anus was excoriated, and she experienced
symptoms similar to dysentery—severe diarrhea with either blood or mucus
in the feces. As many victims of rape do, she kept the tragic event hidden until
her body revealed the secrets she had held on to in silence.[1] The girl's health
continued to deteriorate quickly, and her owner summoned Dr. R. S. Bailey to
treat her. After Bailey's examination, the young girl revealed the details of her
rape, identified her rapist, and told the doctor that he "had since absconded."[2]

The sexual exploitation of enslaved women often worked in tandem with
physicians' medical explorations and publications that medicalized sexual assaults and their physical effects on women. In an effort to illustrate this claim,
this chapter draws on several oral histories of former slaves, medical case narratives, slave owners' personal papers, and judicial cases. In the case of Dr. Bailey's patient, her life is representative of the harrowing experiences that many
female slaves endured. This black girl, who was never safe from either black

or white male intrusion, shows how deeply sex, slavery, and medicine were entangled in nineteenth-century America. Black women's rapes, which were private occurrences, were publicized when members of the slave community reported illnesses to one another, owners, and doctors. Additionally, doctors created professional spaces such as medical journals, teaching hospitals, and colleges where the physical symptoms of these assaults were medicalized. The publication of slave women's rapes in medical writings allowed doctors to learn how to respond to the physical symptoms of sexual assault, such as pregnancy, infertility, venereal disease, and damaged reproductive organs.

Thus when medical men like Dr. Bailey prescribed chemically based medicines for their patients, they were applying the pharmaceutical training many American doctors received in medical colleges. In the case of Bailey's young patient, he gave her a mixture of 3.58 grams of crushed cinchon (an ingredient used to make quinine), 1.79 grams of saltpeter (potassium nitrate), and 2 grams of pulverized opium to treat her symptoms.[3] Cinchon aided nausea, opium led to constipation, and saltpeter helped to ease painful urination. Bailey may have included saltpeter in his prescription because American doctors had been giving the medicine to patients suffering from venereal diseases such as gonorrhea and syphilis since the beginning of the century. A common symptom of gonorrhea and syphilis was urethritis, the medical term for an inflammation of the urethra that causes difficult urination.[4] Most importantly, Bailey pathologized rape and also included black women and girls as victims of rape in a leading medical journal published in a state where they were not legally protected from sexual assault.

Conversely, members of the slave community who lived alongside the victim, particularly black women, would certainly have recognized that the girl had been raped and attempted to comfort her after such a traumatic event. Although Bailey's journal article is silent on what actions black women took to care for this victim, historical literature on slavery offers abundant examples of the maltreatment young black rape victims received from their owners, mistresses, and doctors. The following case highlights the danger black girls faced from white women who discovered their husbands' sexual abuse of female slaves. Thirteen-year-old Maria's mistress caught her in bed with her husband, the girl's master. Upon discovery, the master escaped, and the mistress beat Maria and later had her imprisoned in a smokehouse for two weeks. Older enslaved women pleaded of behalf of the teen girl but were unable to convince their mistress of Maria's victimization.[5] Unlike Maria, Bailey's young enslaved patient was not only regarded as a victim of a brutal rape but also given medical treatment. Sadly, despite the doctor's care and the outpouring of support she received from her community, the girl "died soon after" the rape and subsequent medical intervention made to save her.[6] Both her medical case and her death function as a potent reminder of the complexities of sex, slavery, and medicine in the antebellum South for young black girls and women.

Acclaimed ex-slave memoirist and abolitionist Harriet Jacobs wrote, "The secrets of slavery are concealed like those of the Inquisition."[7] Jacobs used a stark metaphor to describe the horrors she had experienced as an enslaved woman. She wrote that she lived "twenty-one years in that cage of obscene birds" while under the auspices of her master.[8] In this phrase, Jacobs captured the panic that black women faced as they were subjected to the whims of masters who were often "obscene" in their interactions with black women.

The sexual abuse of black women was also an intraracial problem. Scholarly discussions of enslaved men's rape of black girls and women have not been entirely muted; however, scholars need to more fully examine intraracial sexual abuse within slave communities. Two other sites that reveal the inner sexual lives of enslaved women are nineteenth-century medical journals and judicial court records. These sources show how physicians and justices treated intraracial sexual violence within enslaved communities. Enslaved women and girls were vulnerable to attack from white and black men with whom they came into contact. Black women had not only to contend with men who preyed on them but also to fight against the ugly stereotypes that many American men, regardless of race, held about them as wanton seductresses. Robert Smalls, who was born enslaved and later became Reconstruction-era South Carolina's most famous black senator, offered his views on black women's sexual promiscuity to an American Freedmen's Inquiry Commission member after the Civil War. When his interviewer asked Smalls whether black women were full of lust, he answered affirmatively. Smalls also stated, "[Black women] do not consider intercourse an evil thing. This intercourse is principally with white men with whom they would rather have intercourse than with their own color. The majority of the young girls will for money. . . . as young as twelve years."[9] Although the scholarship is slim on this topic, Robert Smalls's views on black women's lustfulness and their supposed preference for engaging in interracial sex for profit, postwar, without regard for their physical and emotional well-being, chastity, and reputations indicate that the sexual terrain for enslaved girls and women was paved with steep hills. Ideologies are formed over time, and Robert Smalls's beliefs probably did not originate solely in the post-1865 racial milieu but were formed in the age of slavery, when messages about black women's lasciviousness went unchallenged.

Enslaved women, whose voices have been muted in medical writings, still managed to name and articulate fully their pain. Some of these women courageously informed doctors in explicit language about their sexual abuse. In

1824, an unidentified enslaved midwife informed Dr. John P. Harrison that her enslaved parturient patient, "A.P.," had been raped and impregnated by a young white man.[10] Harrison, however, did not believe the midwife's account. He wrote in an article published in the *American Journal of Medical Sciences* that no white man would be attracted to a black slave woman who was depicted as a "short, thick-built, chubby creature, with a large head and neck."[11] The crime of rape did not exist for black women during this era. Yet Harrison included the midwife's claim, one he negated, that her patient and fellow slave A.P. had been violated sexually, in the journal article. The midwife might not have been aware of legal statutes concerning rape and black women, but she disclosed all the facts of A.P.'s medical case, which was exacerbated by the violent rape she had experienced.

Bondwomen experienced rape and other types of violent sexual assault frequently. The belief that black women were lascivious was so firmly entrenched in the white psyche that some southern states like South Carolina and Mississippi declared black women could not be raped despite the fact that slave children with white fathers were scattered all over the South. In a famous 1859 court ruling, a Mississippi court declared, "The crime of rape does not exist in this State between African slaves. . . . Their intercourse is promiscuous, and the violation of a female slave would be a mere assault and battery."[12] Celia, a nineteen-year-old Missouri slave woman who had been raped by her owner for five years, murdered him after he entered her cabin to have sex. Her attorneys used a Missouri honor code in her case, arguing that Celia defended her honor against her owner through the use of deadly force. She lost the case and was executed because honor was not a privilege that black and enslaved women could access.[13]

Returning to A.P.'s case, an easy comparison can be drawn between black women's medical experiences and the physical and emotional impact of the kinds of intense physical labor they performed, especially while pregnant. Surely A.P. had to have experienced emotions ranging from anger and frustration to depression and shame because of her treatment by white southern men. The publication of her medical case in a leading medical journal sent a message about black women's honesty, attractiveness, and physicality. Additionally, enslaved women had to contend with the emotional pain caused by rape, disapproving doctors, and difficult pregnancies. Last, for pregnant enslaved women such as A.P., they were also beset by the constant threat that pregnancy and childbirth created: the possibility either they or their babies would die.[14]

What these cases illuminate is that although medicine and law were both sites where "race was made," U.S. medical discourse was capacious enough to recognize enslaved women's rape even when the law did not acknowledge their sexual abuse. One reason for this disparity is that doctors who treated the enslaved, especially women and girls, were much more transparent about describing the physical and sometimes psychological effects of rape because they could medicalize it. The courts, in contrast, did not consider the traumatic impact of black women's rape because of the prevalent ideologies about black women's immorality, and they were interested almost solely in the possible loss of the slave owner's property. The sociopolitical world of antebellum-era slavery and medicine further ensured that enslaved black women would continue to be regarded as "superbodies."

The rape of enslaved women and girls was a component that aided in the continual debasement of black women in American society. Unsurprisingly, black women and girls were denied legal protection by southern states. Historian Sharon Block has argued in her work on rape in early America that for enslaved girls and women, "continuing sexual abuse was often a fact of life." Additionally, few legal mechanisms existed to protect enslaved girls and women from rape, and this "lack of recourse greatly affected their reaction to sexual attacks."[15] A famous court case that took place in Mississippi in 1859 highlights quite boldly how white people considered rape an oxymoron for black women in early America. The state's court dismissed rape charges against an enslaved man named George involving the rape of a ten-year-old enslaved girl. The judge further declared, "The crime of rape does not exist in this State between African slaves."[16] The state later overturned the ruling and created a law that allowed a "negro" or "mulatto" enslaved child under the age of twelve to have legal protection as a victim of rape.[17]

Whether southern legal systems acknowledged the rape of enslaved women and girls or not, the fact remained that this vulnerable population, their owners, and medical doctors had to confront the physical, medical, and psychic realities of rape in enslaved black women's lives. Slaves were forbidden autonomous mobility; it was illegal without the owner's consent, so most rape victims stayed put. Thus most enslaved girls and women suffered the physical wounds and illnesses brought on by their sexual assaults in sight of their rapists, and there are medical journal articles that reflect this historical fact.

Alongside women in slave communities who provided healing according to the "relational vision of health" that Sharla Fett articulates, a view of healing that was both sacred and secular, medical doctors administered curative work but relied almost exclusively on chemical medicine to heal black women.[18] Black women healers, on the other hand, practiced a relational vision of health anchored in a belief that their healing would be left not solely to human beings but to God and their ancestors. Dreams and signs were just as relevant as any medicine a doctor prescribed, even more so in many slave communities.

The antebellum era was a pivotal moment in the lives of both enslaved black women and white medical men because the landscape for professional women's health care was in flux. There was an emergent class of male midwives, professed experts in gynecology, and also doctors who began to treat women exclusively; their numbers were small but growing. The following case sheds light on the changes that were occurring. While Fanny, a middle-aged slave, was giving birth, both she and the baby she delivered died under Dr. John A. Wragg's care. According to the doctor's subsequent article in the *Southern Journal of Medicine and Pharmacy*, before his arrival a Savannah, Georgia, plantation "Negro" midwife had treated Fanny. Wragg also wrote that the enslaved midwife's assessment of Fanny's condition must "be taken with some degree of caution." He did add, however, that the midwife's story should be thought of as "tolerably accurate and trustworthy" because she was intelligent.[19] Wragg then posed a question that became foundational for how white medical doctors should assess enslaved black women's healing work, even tolerably "intelligent" ones. He asked readers, "Could, or rather would the life of this woman have been saved, had a physician been called in earlier?"[20] His question indicates a shift from the idea and practice that women were the natural caretakers of pregnant women to one where medical men should attend to all births.

The nature of nineteenth-century medicine was mainly exploratory; searching for the root cause of a medical condition, however, especially surgically based research in gynecological medicine, could be exceedingly dangerous for enslaved patients who were subjected to such operations. Once medical training moved from an apprenticeship culture to one that was more scientifically based in the 1800s, medical research became more important to doctors. During the seventeenth and eighteenth centuries, according to Abraham Flexner's influential 1910 report on medical education, medical schools "existed as a supplement to the apprenticeship system."[21]

As gynecology grew, doctors wrote about nearly every manner of women's diseases and conditions in medical journals, thereby extending the reach of medical education beyond schools. As these men engaged in finding cures for women's reproductive illnesses, some surgically based, like the repair of vesico-vaginal fistulae, gynecological medical experimentation increased, especially on enslaved women. In the South, white doctors had a vulnerable and accessible black population on which they could perform operations and test cures. The widely held belief that black women suffered from gynecological diseases disproportionately encouraged such experimentation.[22] Historian William Dosite Postell cites an example of such notions, observing that southern doctors believed that "uterine troubles were of common occurrence among slave women."[23]

Another manifestation of the distinctions that doctors made between the sexuality of black women and that of white women is the different protocol they followed during physical examinations, based on the patient's race. Determining the source of gynecological conditions required that doctors examine black women's naked bodies, even though the practice was rare in medical circles for white women. Medical men generally did not gaze upon their white female patients' once they had disrobed except during emergencies. In contrast, white physicians generally shared the assumption that black women were immodest about the display of their bodies, and medical doctors examined black women's breasts, stomachs, and genitalia without reserve. The history of enslaved black women's handling by white men in the Americas began with the institutionalization of slavery during the early sixteenth century and continued into the nineteenth century. Later, medical doctors were included in the evaluation process and began to examine black women in southern slave markets.[24] Concurrently, as gynecology developed and American medicine was formalized, enslaved women's examinations became part and parcel of doctors' medical work as they assessed black women's economic value.

In 1825, Dr. Finley, of Charleston, South Carolina, published an article that detailed his examination of a bondwoman in her midforties who was "menstruating from her mammae."[25] Although Finley did not indicate whether the enslaved woman's condition was unique, he found it interesting enough to share the case with his peers. He wrote that his patient could not provide an exact date when the discharges had begun; further, she claimed ignorance about the nature of her nipple bleeding. She informed Finley that she suffered pain in her side, experienced anal bleeding, and was fatigued. She stated that above all she wanted to be relieved from her agony. Paradoxically, despite all the symptoms that the enslaved woman shared with Finley, he was unable to diagnose the cause of her condition. He seems not to have considered whether the patient had cancer, a tumor, or even a cyst. Rather, Finley determined that his black patient could experience not only a normal menstrual cycle but also an abnormal one located in her "menstruating breast."[26] The unnamed enslaved patient became another model of black female abnormality, the epitome of the "medical superbody." In her case, her period could be experienced not only in her uterus and ovaries but also in her breast. Although she was not described as freakish, it was clear that Finley regarded her condition as beyond the scope of a "normal" women's disease.

In response to her ailment, Finley petitioned other "professional gentleman of this city" to provide him with information concerning her illness in the *Carolina Journal of Medicine, Science, and Agriculture*.[27] He promised that, in return for the medical services he would render to the enslaved patient, he would allow his colleagues to experiment on the bondwoman for pedagogical purposes. As his requests reveal, the slave woman's recovery was less critical to the attending physician than the medical lessons he and his colleagues could possibly glean from an observation of her "menstruating" breasts.[28]

James Marion Sims operated as both a doctor and a slave owner. Dr. Sims believed that the survival of black slave women depended on his medical expertise; however, his career proved that the opposite was true: Sims depended on enslaved black women's bodies to discover cures for vesico-vaginal fistulae and perfect surgical instruments such as the duckbilled speculum, achievements that were responsible for his global status as a pioneering gynecological surgeon. As the philosopher Georg Wilhelm Friedrich Hegel observed in *The Phenomenology of Mind*, "The master relates himself to the bondsman immediately through independent existence, for that is precisely what keeps the bondsman in thrall; it is his chain."[29] The enslaved women Sims treated, however, possessed bodies and lives that were not contingent upon the advancement of gynecology. Black women could and did conceive of themselves and their worth without the inclusion of white men.

Black women often continued their midwifery work even after slavery ended, demonstrating they did not want white men's permission, intrusion, and instruction to perform medical work that they believed they had mastered. While enslaved, Mildred Graves labored for decades as a nurse and midwife in Hanover, Virginia, for her owner, Mr. Tinsley. Graves serviced both black and white women because of her reputation as an exemplary accoucheur and "doctoring woman." Despite her position, Graves suffered ridicule and shameful debasement by white doctors. She remembered a particularly traumatic episode when her owner sent her to assist Mrs. Leake, a pregnant white patient who was experiencing a protracted labor. Upon reaching Leake, Graves encountered two doctors from Richmond there to assist in the child's delivery. The doctors informed Graves that they were unable to help Leake. Graves responded, "I could bring her 'roun'." As the bondwoman later recalled, the doctors "laugh at me an' say, 'Get back, darkie. We mean business an' don' wont any witch doctors or hoodoo stuff.'"[30] Leake, however, insisted that Graves deliver her baby, and the midwife did so successfully. Mildred Graves reported defiantly that the doctors who condemned her "said many praise fer [her]."[31]

The enslaved Graves courageously dealt with the doctors' general hostility toward her race, gender, and enslaved status, their mocking of her African-based medicinal knowledge, and their dismissal of her skill set. The obstetrical case allowed her to transcend, momentarily, the marked racial and gendered boundaries set for her in a racially stratified society. Though her white patient served as the impetus for the exchange to occur, the woman's delivery was as a potent reminder that enslaved doctoring women could rarely escape the white gaze and condemnation.[32]

Another site where enslaved women and white men, doctors and slave owners alike, had contested relations was the area of slave family planning. The sexual abuse that enslaved women endured certainly exacted a toll on their bodies and psyches, but the prospect of becoming mothers could often serve as a powerful antidote to their suffering. Sometimes women received gifts as rewards for "breeding" children. During Mary Reynolds's enslavement, she recalled her owner's promise to give every woman on the plantation who birthed twins within a year's time "a outfittin' of clothes for the twins and a double warm blanket."[33] The owner's incentive for the women to bear twins, as if they could will themselves to deliver multiple children during a birthing session, emphasizes how ignorant some men were about reproduction. Also, the owner's promise of an especially warm blanket reveals the scarcity of these essential items for pregnant enslaved women.

Some bondwomen, like Martha Bradley, struck out at white men who offended them by attempting to suggest they enter into sexual unions. Bradley shared a story with her interviewer: "One day I was working in the field, and the overseer he come round and say somep'n to me had no business say. I took my hoe and knocked him plumb down. . . . I say to Marster Lucas what that overseer say to me and Marster Lucas didn't hit me no more."[34] Her case was highly unusual because of the counternarrative of victimization it provides but also because of the response of her master, who surprisingly ceased whipping her upon learning of the overseer's transgression. Feminist scholar Saidiya V. Hartman posits, "The enslaved is legally unable to give consent or offer resistance, she is presumed to be always willing."[35] Yet Bradley's reaction to Lucas informs scholars that some enslaved women, if provoked, readily used violence as a weapon to protect themselves against men who insulted their moral sensibilities by acting on the assumption that black women wanted to sleep with them. More broadly, historian Stephanie Camp has argued that "for bondswomen . . . intimate entities such as the body and the home were instruments of both domination and resistance."[36]

Martha Bradley's story elucidates the disparate methods some enslaved women employed to claim honor for themselves as protection against sexual dominance and exploitation by men, who often viewed them as hypersexualized. Bradley's recollection of this event to a government worker illustrates two major considerations: First, her case emphasizes that some whites, like Martha's owner, might have believed that black women could indeed possess honor in their interactions with white men. Second, one can speculate that Bradley offered this story to underscore the meaning she gave to herself in ways that whites did not.

This latter point conveys the role of agency that some formerly enslaved persons sought to insert in the historical record, which reminds us of the importance of historical memory. The übersexuality that white society attributed to the black woman's body has origins that date back centuries. Winthrop Jordan cites an instance of this historical reality, writing, "By forging a sexual link between Negroes and apes, . . . Englishmen were able to give vent to their feelings that Negroes were a lewd, lascivious, and wanton people."[37]

Acts of resistance such as Bradley's offer us insight into the ways that enslaved women actively sought authority over their lives. Independently choosing and maintaining loving relationships with black men was one of the ways black women resisted white control over the most intimate and personal parts of their lives. Lucy Ann Dunn, a North Carolina enslaved woman, articulated powerfully the love she had for her husband, Jim Dunn, and their eight children. Dunn told her interviewer, "We lived together fifty-five years and . . . I loved him durin' life and . . . though he's been dead for twelve years . . . I want to go to Jim . . . when I smell honeysuckles or see a yellow moon."[38] Mrs. Dunn's memories shine a light on the importance of black male and female romantic partnerships during slavery. Also, having children was essential for black women and the black men they loved because it cemented notions of family and self even on a shaky foundation.

Bondwomen's actions and testimonies about reproduction and parenting suggest that some enslaved women defined the terms under which they would both birth and parent "their" children." For example, Mrs. James Seward's sister, also an enslaved mother, claimed ownership of herself and her infant child in direct defiance of her owner's wishes. When the toddler began to walk, her master sold the child. Seward explained that her sister "went and got it [her child]" after the sale was finalized.[39] Her act of defiance alerted her master that her position as the baby's mother would trump any decision he made. Further, she proved she would intervene in the child's life at her discretion.

For those bondwomen who resisted the reproductive control of white men, planned pregnancies were a form of "womb liberation" especially when supportive black midwives offered them prenatal care and used less-intrusive medical treatments. Dellie Lewis, whose grandmother served as a plantation midwife, explained that her grandmother typically gave enslaved obstetrical patients "cloves and whiskey to ease the pain."[40] As gynecology developed, however, white men's intrusion into black women's reproductive lives became even more prominent. The contours of enslavement did not grant bondwomen the liberty to prevent physicians from performing risky experimental surgeries on them or giving them dangerous drugs for medical complications that often arose in delivery.

The following case elucidates this point. In August 1819, Nanny, a Columbia, South Carolina, enslaved woman, lay in agony for sixty hours because she was unable to give birth naturally. Despite the presence of a slave midwife, her labor could not be induced. Afraid that Nanny and her child would die, the midwife called Dr. Charles Atkins to intervene in this obstetrical case. After Nanny was examined, she underwent emergency surgeries on her bladder, ruptured cervix, and vagina. She endured the surgeries over a two-day period. Nanny was a high-risk obstetric and gynecologic patient because she was carrying twins who had died in utero. Her doctor removed one stillborn child by "hand art" and the other, the second day, with his surgical blade. As risky as antebellum-era surgeries were, Nanny amazingly survived the procedures.[41] Although Nanny represents many antebellum-era enslaved women who lost children during childbirth, the early publication of her medical experiences was not so common.

The nineteenth century was a watershed era in American gynecologic medicine. White men entered a field that had been dominated by women for millennia, but these men also pioneered surgical advances that repaired obstetrical fistulae, removed diseased ovaries, and performed successful cesarean section operations. In the South, as discussed earlier, enslaved women were disproportionately represented in these early surgical experiments. Physicians worked on them in their homes, hospitals, and classrooms. As doctors wrote about black women's diseases and bodies, their colleagues, perhaps inadvertently, learned how to think about and treat black women from medical journal articles. Doctors created a metanarrative about race, ability, and gender that centered on "black" women. This metanarrative might have been peppered with technical jargon about medical procedures, but their writings unquestionably offered an early "technology" of race through medicine. The technology of race was certainly employed in medical journals and the pedagogical framework of medical training taught in medical hospitals because it, as Evelyn Brooks Higginbotham argues, "signif[ied] the elaboration and implementation of discourses (classificatory and evaluative) in order to maintain the survival and hegemony of one group over another."[42] The metanarrative was deeply nuanced not because of its foundation in the politics of race and medical knowledge, always a contentious issue in antebellum America, but rather because much of the metanarrative included enslaved people's voices. When doctors chose to include their voices in medical literature, their testimony revealed deep fissures in the ideology of white Southern paternalism and black people's acceptance of this so-called benevolence. In numerous medical case narratives, doctors would write about the soundness and strength that black people possessed despite their illnesses and the ease with which black patients managed pain. Yet, in the same narratives, contradictions appeared that revealed black patients' frailties and pains. In Nanny's case, enslaved men and women intervened on her behalf because they witnessed the wasting away of her physical strength and vitality taking place because she "bred" so often.

The narrative of Nanny's medical case exposed the concerns of the enslaved men and women from her community. They informed Dr. Atkins of their feelings about Nanny's physical frailty due to her seven former pregnancies.[43] They declared Nanny should have never been allowed to "breed" because her body was "too delicate." Notwithstanding Nanny's fragility, at least according to the black plantation community, her final prognosis was positive, according to Dr. Atkins. She recovered, having survived a harrowing physical ordeal, and became infertile, a condition that most probably decreased her economic value. Historian Marie Jenkins Schwartz has noted the importance of reproductive health for both the enslaved woman and her master during the antebellum era. She asserts, "A dual approach to the management of women's health developed on Southern plantations."[44] Although black enslaved women and their white male owners were invested in maintaining black women's gynecological health, their reasons and methods varied. Nanny's case demonstrates the saliency of Jenkins Schwartz's argument because it demonstrates how physicians, like slave owners, were similarly invested in highlighting black women's "difference" and thus their "inferiority" to white women. Despite her extensive surgeries, seven in all, Nanny's quick recovery postsurgery and subsequent good health and strength seemed to prove the hardiness of black women, especially those "fit" for labor like bondwomen.

American medicine developed under the expansive influence of European scientific racism. As a consequence, early gynecologists demonstrated their medical knowledge through their treatment of and writings about enslaved women as gynecological patients who purportedly felt little or no pain as they underwent invasive surgical procedures.[45] Antebellum-era doctors continued the American tradition of reinforcing prevailing racial stereotypes about "black" women through their writings. These men recognized the importance of medical journals, especially as the field became more legitimized.

As the field of gynecology emerged, enslaved women had to learn to manage growing medical intrusions into their sexual lives, interference that often made them ill. Enslaved women were often forced to have intercourse with men whom their owners chose for them to "marry." In an interview years after she was freed, Marriah Hines noted that her master had married her to a man of his choosing, and she had "five chullun by him."[46] In cases where women birthed children from rape or were forced to rear children whom they had not borne, they faced a host of complex issues. More amazingly, how did enslaved women negotiate their paths inside the brutal terrain of slavery and maintain a firm hold on their sanity? Bondwomen's insistence on exercising reproductive autonomy helped form what might be called a liberation doctrine, one that stressed their humanity, strength, resiliency, and intelligence. Their metalanguage, "language that supersedes multiple categories of difference," was contained within their acts of resistance and survival.[47]

When Marriah Hines mentioned that her owner married her to a man for whom she bore five children, she also acknowledged that she learned to love and celebrate him. Hines stated that her husband was "one of the best colored man in the world."[48] The larger issue of brutality cannot be overstated when we examine how masters took away enslaved people's right to choose who they desired romantically. Yet even in the context of Hines's dehumanization, she chose to celebrate her husband's manhood and her love for him. Black women's ability to love romantic partners forced on them was very similar to their choosing to love children resulting from rape or to nurture those they were forced to raise after the children's parents had been sold away. Bond-women's resistance must be read as a central theme critical to understanding the totality of their lives even as they lived within the restrictive contours of slavery and professional medicine. Unfortunately, although gynecologists sometimes included enslaved women's words in medical narratives, their metanarrative of race and medicine did not take into full account black women's metalanguage of race. Thus historians of slavery and medicine must continue to examine and interpret how enslaved women responded to the medical treatments and behavior of doctors and slave owners, keeping in mind that these sources were authored solely by white men.[49]

Metanarratives about black women's bodies, health, and responses to white people's medical interventions also crossed gender lines. White plantation women sometimes recorded how black women responded to their illnesses and treatments in their personal writings. Noted diarist and former Georgia plantation mistress, the English-born actress Frances Kemble detailed how her husband, Pierce Butler, routinely treated sick bondwomen on his plantation. Kemble documented a troubling incident that involved Teresa, a woman they owned. She wrote, "With an almost savage vehemence of gesticulation . . . [Teresa] tore her scanty clothing, and exhibited a spectacle . . . which inconceivably shocked and sickened. . . . These are natural results, inevitable and irremediable ones, of improper treatment of the female frame."[50] Kemble sympathized with Teresa's pain but also expressed her simultaneous amazement and repulsion at the woman's appearance and behavior. Equally distressing to Kemble was her husband's ability to carry on his daily duties with neither interruption nor concern for Teresa. Slavery created a space where white people could witness the most horrific acts of sheer brutality and viciousness against other humans, and without a misstep, they could make love, go to church, and kiss their children good night.

Parthena Rollins, an ex-slave from Kentucky, experienced the macabre nature of slavery's brutality and hesitated to discuss her experiences under the institution nearly seven decades after its abolishment. She shared that the abuses she and other slaves suffered in bondage by stating plainly to her white interviewer that what black slaves endured "would make your hairs stand on ends."[51] Rollins recalled the murder of an enslaved infant before its mother. Slave traders came ready to purchase the seemingly robust and strong young mother; however, they were adamant about not buying her baby. The woman's owner, wanting to make a sale, quickly beat the child until it died.[52] After her sale, the slave woman began to have seizures. According to Rollins, the woman's "fits" were brought on by her child's cruel murder. In another act of cruelty, her new master refused to pay the costs involved in providing the bereaved mother with necessary medical treatment and instead returned the woman to her former owner and asked for a full refund. Rollins declared finally, "She could hardly talk of the happenings of the early days because of the awful things her folks had to go through."[53]

Although enslaved mothers were aware that they could be sold away from their children, they were not prepared to deal with the murder of their offspring and the trauma following these painful occurrences. Although Rollins's example is rare, it is deeply significant because of its bold example of black women's intersecting experiences with sexuality, reproduction, economic value, death, and medicine.

Enslaved mothers often went to great lengths to protect their children from the excessive violence of slave owners and overseers. In doing so, these bondwomen arguably fashioned a form of honor unique to their experiences as reproductive laborers. Fannie Moore offered a moving testimony of maternal protection, describing the punishments that her mother would often suffer to shield her children from the brutality of the plantation overseer. Speaking of her mother with pride, Moore stated, "She stan' up fo' her chillun tho'. De ol overseeah he hate my mammy, case she fight him for beatin' her chillun. Why she git more whuppings for dat den anythin' else. She hab twelve chillun."[54] As the reaction of Moore's mother reveals, some enslaved women were willing to attack white men for viciously abusing their children, regardless of the violence inflicted on their own bodies.

The narrative of Canadian refugee Mrs. John Little provides a deeper view of how enslaved women fought back through silence, suffering, and ultimately cunning. She shared her story of being a member of a contingent of Virginia slaves who crafted an escape plan, which initially failed because of the betrayal of a group member. For the two women involved, sex and reproduction were connected to their punishments when caught. Mrs. Little stated, "The master made a remark to the overseer about my shape. Before striking me, master questioned me about the girl. . . . I only knew that she had been with child, and that now she was not, but I did not tell them even of that. I was ashamed of my situation, they remarking upon me."[55] The other woman Mrs. Little mentioned received an abortion from an enslaved woman who was made aware of their escape plan. Perhaps it was an enslaved midwife who provided Little's comrade with the abortion, but all the women decided it was the most appropriate medical action to take before they escaped.

The work of renowned natural scientist Louis Agassiz stands as a testament to how black women lacked control of their bodies and images in almost every conceivable way. Drana was an enslaved South Carolinian whose father was Congo born. Agassiz commissioned South Carolina daguerreotypist J. T. Zealy to capture Drana's image for observation and educational purposes. Agassiz was a firm believer in polygenism, the theory that racial groups did not share a common ancestor as the Bible asserted, and these pictures would help to prove the validity of his belief.[56] Drana was photographed both frontally and sideways with her breasts bared. It was clear that these daguerreotypes were meant to document black people as scientific specimens, wholly distinct from white people. Figure 3.1 is a daguerreotype taken in 1850 when the emergence of Americans interest in scientific racism had crystallized with the emergence of the American school of ethnology, advanced by physicians Samuel Cartwright and Josiah Nott and early ethnologist Samuel Morton, among others.[57] The American school was decidedly antiblack.

In slavery and in the annals of antebellum-era medical education, the representations of and writings about the black female body had been used to shame black people. Further, these writings situated black women as the diametric opposite of white women, who, though still viewed as the abnormal sex, were considered virginal and virtuous. Slave owners and medical doctors inscribed the enslaved black female body not only to reflect gendered notions of racial resiliency but also to aid in the commodification of slavery. Enslaved women's anatomies would determine if an owner's wealth increased through her sale or whether a physician's good reputation stayed intact, and her fertility could supposedly be determined by the appearance of her reproductive organs. In the North, however, another dispossessed group of women shared similar medical

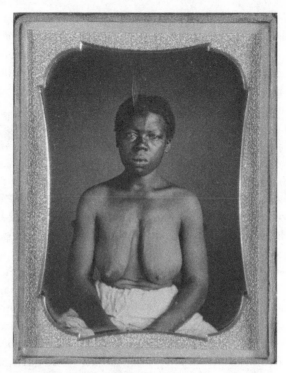

FIGURE 3.1. Daguerreotype of Drana, a South Carolina slave,
by J. T. Zealy, commissioned by Louis Agassiz, 1850.
Courtesy of the Peabody Museum of Archaeology and Ethnology,
Photographic Archives Collection, Harvard University.

and racialized experiences: poor Irish immigrant women. If there was one thing
that linked the medical experiences of enslaved and Irish women, it was the notion that blackness, the ultimate mark of difference and inferiority in America,
could be mapped onto bodies that were deemed degraded. Between 1800 and
1865, an important historical period in the development of modern gynecology
and obstetrics, medical and scientific research on the racialized body reached
its apogee.

CHAPTER FOUR

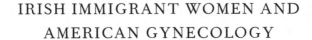

IRISH IMMIGRANT WOMEN AND AMERICAN GYNECOLOGY

Oh brave, brave Irish girls,
We well might call you brave
Should the least of all your perils
The Stormy ocean waves.

—James Connally, *Labour in Ireland*

Accordingly it is found, that the patients generally are irregular
and careless in their attendance, and pay but little attention
to direction. The greater part are extremely ignorant.

—William Buell, writing on the behavior of his
poor Irish immigrant patients

THE GYNECOLOGICAL EXPERIENCES OF IRISH IMMIGRANT WOMEN IN America began following the transatlantic voyages they took after they fled Ireland because of a potato famine that left them and their nation hungry and desperate. Their sexual exploitation, however, began before these ships reached their destination. Like African women who were forced to board slave ships for the Americas three centuries earlier, nineteenth-century Irish immigrant women also suffered sexual abuses on "coffin ships," so named because of the number of people who died during oceanic voyages to America. The thousands of Irish women headed to the United States were young, alone, and unprotected as they traveled aboard these vessels. For those women who were sexually abused, the boats represented floating prisons where they were unable to escape the sexual violence inflicted on them. The notes and published writings of ship captains, newspaper reporters, and others who chronicled the Irish immigrant seaboard experience described the collective sufferings that both male and female immigrants endured. While they did not emphasize sexual assaults, they compared the atrocities the Irish experienced with those that West African captives had undergone on slave ships. A March 10, 1847, article published in the *Cork Examiner* detailed conditions aboard the *Medemseh*, a ship carrying Irish passengers to New York City. The author wrote, "It reflects disgrace upon the regulations of the Government that creatures in this condition should be suffered to proceed to sea, with no other dependence against a long and enfeebling voyage than the kindness of persons whose treatment of their passengers, on an average, is hardly less brutal than that experienced from the masters of slave-ships."[1]

More broadly, maritime travel was intimately connected to medicine because of the physical examinations passengers underwent when they arrived in the United States. When the ships reached their destinations, doctors examined the surviving passengers' bodies for deformities, diseases, and perceived abnormalities. Before the 1880s, few governmental and social agencies devoted considerable resources to assessing who met the criteria for "unfit immigrants." In addition, women with gynecological disorders might have been able to escape examination because their illnesses were sometimes internal rather than external. Further, the journal articles that doctors wrote about Irish immigrant women, which detailed their medical practices and thoughts, helped to create the foundation for racist laws that colored the Irish as not quite white and sometimes placed them alongside black people as biological models for racial inferiority.[2] As such, immigration became enmeshed in nineteenth-century systems of social control, just as the institution of slavery concerned discipline, surveillance, and ultimately control. For this reason, the later development of modern American gynecology can no more be disentangled from Irish immigration than it can be separated from its roots in slavery.

One year after the *Cork Examiner* reported on the atrocities committed aboard the *Medemseh*, well-known archbishop John Hughes wrote a passionate letter to Irish American leader Robert Emmet about the number of sexual assaults committed against Irish women aboard these U.S.-bound ships. Cloaked in the restrained Victorian language of the day, Archbishop Hughes commented on the different set of protections that were needed in America for Irish women. Hughes stated, "The protection of a shield" was not necessary in Ireland because Irish women allegedly did not experience this kind of sexual violence at home.[3] Yet, for "pure, innocent" Irish women who were supposedly ignorant of the "snares of the world, and the dangers to which poverty and inexperience would expose them in a foreign land," a mighty shield was necessary.[4]

As Irish women landed in American port cities, even more "snares" awaited them. They entered the country as members of the largest European immigrant group to live in major cities, and they faced a bleak economic landscape.[5] Job options were limited, and Irish women worked physically challenging, low-wage jobs such as factory labor, trash collection, and domestic service that were often dangerous and unhealthy. Although the Irish immigrant women were free laborers, historians like Hasia Diner, Alan Kraut, and Kevin Kelly have argued that thousands of these women became enmeshed in an antebellum labor system that was static and reduced them to wage slavery. Without financial stability, Irish women were unable to protect themselves against many of the dangers that urban women faced, including overcrowded and unsanitary housing, violence, and prostitution. Further, until the last half of the century, poor Irish women often stood outside the protective barriers accessible to native-born white women. For example, the protection of white women's sexuality and reproduction had been a basic feature of early British colonialism, American nationalism, and white supremacy since the seventeenth century, when the first laws evolved that distinguished blackness from whiteness. By the 1800s, a famous article in London's popular magazine *Punch*, "The Missing Link," cautioned readers to protect themselves against an Irish "creature manifestly between the Gorilla and the Negro."[6] Finally, in 1860, political leaders drafted a congressional act designed "to regulate the carriage of passengers in steamships and other vessels, for the better protection of female passengers."[7] This act represented the wide-ranging shield that Archbishop Hughes wanted for Irish victims of sexual violence. While this law stopped neither shipboard rapes nor sexual assaults on land, it did codify whiteness for Irish women who had experienced American anti-Irish discrimination.

The most intimate details of poor Irish immigrant women's medical and reproductive lives could not escape public discourse, largely because social welfare and reform issues focused on immigrants in the northeastern cities where most of these women lived. Comparable to southern enslaved women whose bodies fueled the advancement of the field, Irish-born women's bodies helped to create a nascent urban social-welfare system and to a lesser degree, maintained American gynecology as a dynamic branch of medicine.

One group in particular held special interest for men interested in collecting statistical data and gaining a better understanding of sexuality, criminality, behavior, and race: Irish prostitutes. Lacking skills, family support, and opportunities, and having been sexually abused on ship, many Irish women immigrants turned to prostitution to earn a living. Public health officials, Irish nationalists, Catholic leaders, and government workers were aware of the sustained sexual abuse that Irish women faced at sea and on land. Thus the establishment of hospitals and institutions devoted to Irish women's medical care was an integral component of Irish American community building. More importantly, the institution building that occurred moved Irish-born women closer to middle-class respectability. White northerners, including abolitionists, did not offer free black women who engaged in sex work the kind of brick-and-mortar institutions that were meant to mold them into respectable ladies. Irish immigrant women occupied the bottom rung of the economic ladder alongside black women, yet they still benefited from the existence of an affluent Irish-Catholic community that was concerned about their care. Institutional assistance was especially prominent as the field of gynecology's developed and sex workers, needing medical care, suffered from a number of sexually transmitted infections. It is important to note that not all Irish immigrant women were sex workers or victimized, and some might very well have been sexually liberated in their private lives despite the controlling influence of the church and other charitable institutions.

The notion of owning one's own body loomed large for impoverished Irish immigrant women for many reasons. Many women were forced to sell their bodies to men who claimed possession of them as pimps. Many others worked as little more than wage slaves as domestics, factory workers, and street peddlers, which often meant that their bodies, mobility, and autonomy were at the disposal of their male bosses. Accordingly, Irish women's roles as sex workers (whether assumed to be voluntarily or not) posed a growing social problem for nineteenth-century reformers. Sex work was dangerous, placed women at great risk for contracting sexually transmitted infections, and also marked them as immoral. John Francis Maguire, writing about the entry of the Irish into America, states, "*Innocent and unprotected girls, came consigned to houses of prostitution.*"[8]

Although no comprehensive studies exist that determine how Irish women sex workers contracted sexually transmitted infections (largely because germ theory had not been discovered and infections contracted from sexual contact could be difficult to diagnose), it is likely that many of these infections were caused by sexual violence.

Leading the charge for moral reform was the Catholic Church, which sanctioned the opening of many privately owned hospitals and almshouses. Poor Irish immigrant women used institutions such as New York City's Saint Vincent's Hospital to attend to their spiritual and physical needs. Not only were these institutions medically necessary resources for this immigrant group, but they also served as physical testaments to the desire of Irish people to prove that they were not deviant and, in fact, wanted to improve their condition in America. For the women who used them, the act of choosing where to be treated medically was one of the ways they claimed ownership of their bodies and medical experiences.

In 1850s New York, the Irish Catholic Sisters of Mercy would "nurse the newly arrived so they would be healthy enough to perform hard labor in a few weeks' time."[9] Catholic groups like the Sisters of Mercy, Sisters of the Good Shepherd Convent, and the Sisters of Charity proved indispensable to thousands of Irish-immigrant women. Historian Jean Richardson points out that northern "antebellum hospitals did not profess to cure illnesses, but rather warehoused the poverty-stricken sick" who were either homeless or lived in unsanitary tenements unfit for recovery.[10] In contrast, the Catholic organizations that devoted themselves to caring for Irish immigrant women made every effort to heal them. The House of the Good Shepherd, the charitable outgrowth of the Sisters of the Good Shepherd, was a controversial charitable antebellum organization because of its focus on aiding Irish prostitutes.[11] Prostitutes would use the House of the Good Shepherd when they needed housing and medical attention, "particularly for sexually transmitted diseases."[12]

In 1857, William Sanger, a well-known medical doctor, researched the history of prostitution and sexually transmitted diseases in the city. He published statistically driven scholarship that illustrated the sheer volume of venereal disease cases reported by a range of professionals from New York institutions offering medical services. He noted that as a matter of practice, many physicians treated venereal cases "under some other name" in their official reports.[13] They renamed sexually transmitted diseases because several public dispensaries and hospitals had regulations forbidding the admission of venereal patients. Sanger noted that the trustees at a hospital in a New York sister city, "which receives a yearly grant from public funds, has in its printed rules and regulations: 'No person having "Gonorrhea" or "Syphilis" shall be admitted as a charity patient.'"[14] One can speculate that this hospital's nonadmission policy on syphilitics and those with gonorrhea was predicated on moral beliefs about a person's character based on the sexual nature of these infections. Other facilities such as prison hospitals could not institute discriminatory admittance polices. The census figures of those inmates who were recorded as having "venereal diseases" were far greater than those of most hospitals. As the resident physician at Blackwell's Island, a correctional facility, Sanger found that incarcerated women had higher rates of sexually transmitted infections than those who were not imprisoned. These institutions tended to house a disproportionately large number of Irish immigrant women. In his study, Sanger compiled an index of most of the venereal patients treated in New York City–area hospitals and dispensaries in 1857. Table 4.1 lists the reported figures from hospitals for women patients.

TABLE 4.1 Number of Reproductive and Sexually Transmitted Illnesses in Greater New York City

Institutions	Cases
Penitentiary Hospital, Blackwell's Island	2,090
Almshouse, Blackwell's Island	52
Workhouse, Blackwell's Island	56
Penitentiary, Blackwell's Island	430
Bellevue Hospital, New York	768
Nursery Hospital, Randall's Island	734
New York State Emigrants' Hospital, Ward Island	559
New York Hospital, Broadway	405
New York Dispensary, Centre Street	1,580
Northern Dispensary, Waverly Place	327
Eastern Dispensary, Ludlow Street	630
Demilt Dispensary, Second Avenue	803
Northwestern Dispensary, Eighth Avenue	344
Medical Colleges	207
King's County Hospital, Flatbush, Long Island	311
Brooklyn City Hospital, Brooklyn, Long Island	186
Seaman's Retreat, Staten Island	365
TOTAL	9,847

Source: Sanger, History of Prostitution, 593.

Unfortunately, the statistical data on the medical lives of Irish-immigrant women is scant when compared to the data on enslaved women, and the reliability of these figures is problematic for many reasons. Despite the ambiguity of Sanger's figures on racial identity and disease, they still provide enough information for contextualization. Poor and immigrant communities were frequently overpoliced, and their members were incarcerated more often than the general population. The figures reported do not provide an exact calculation of how many of these patients were Irish born. However, with the disproportionate number of Irish women who were imprisoned because of prostitution, it is likely that a large percentage of these prisoners were of Irish descent. Further, these alarming statistics point to the roles and growing importance of medical professionals who treated women suffering from sexually contracted infections and reveal how poor white women's sexual labor was linked not only to vice but to disease.

Irish immigrants were familiar with dehumanizing descriptions of them that compared them to Africans and apes. In essence, they were used to anti-Irish Anglo racism, and connections were constantly made through public discourse and in the writings generated in the medical and scientific worlds to illustrate the limitations of their whiteness and the relative close ties they had with blackness. As anti-Irish and antiblack racism gained a larger platform, obstetrics and gynecology became another area where white antebellum-era medical men could make claims about gender, difference, and race with scientific authority.

During this same era, the entrance of American gynecology as an emerging medical specialty dependent on women's sick bodies made Irish-born women an attractive patient population for northern-based doctors who had begun to work primarily on women. Some gynecologists like James Marion Sims, who had previously worked within slave communities, extended their surgical work to include Irish women in the charity wards of northern hospitals. For southern migrants like Sims, it was not much of a stretch to treat poor Irish women patients as he had enslaved women because much of the Anglo world's racial science, popular literature, and racially biased views of this group held that Irish women were able to withstand physical pain just as black women could.

The case of Mary Smith, Dr. Sims's first New York State Woman's Hospital patient, exemplifies how poor Irish women had to navigate a medical system in which doctors explained women's biological sicknesses in ways that also gave meaning to women's nature and the world men and women occupied. Medical historian Charles Rosenberg states, "Explaining sickness is too significant— socially and emotionally—for it to be a value free enterprise."[15] Dr. Sims's Woman's Hospital could not be a neutral healing space, for it separated rich women from poor women and endowed only men with the liberty to become experts on women's diseases. When Sims asserted that the New York hospital would become "a place in which [he could] show the world what [he was] capable of doing," he was also claiming that his hospital would serve as a site for his personal and professional aggrandizement.[16]

Mary Smith was an Irish immigrant from western Ireland, the country's poorest region, and had arrived in New York as a single mother and a poor sick woman. She would come to represent thousands of poor Irish immigrant women who were connected to New York City's hospitals. Historian Bernadette McCauley states, "By midcentury, the patient population at city hospitals was overwhelmingly foreign-born. . . . By 1866, more than half the admissions had been born in Ireland."[17] Hospital administrators, some of whom might have harbored nativist sentiments against foreign patients, sometimes created hostile environments for Irish immigrant patients like Mary Smith. One Massachusetts General Hospital trustee member claimed that the Irish, as a group, were ignorant and unappreciative medical patients.[18] He stated, "They cannot appreciate & do not really want, some of those conveniences which would be deemed essential by most of our native citizens." He believed that sick Irish men and women would be more comfortable and appreciative if they were treated in a "cheap building" instead of more expensive and well-maintained hospitals.[19] Living in 1850s New York City, Smith had to have been aware of anti-Irish sentiments held by New Yorkers, and perhaps because the Woman's Hospital was new, she sought services from a hospital that did not have a history of anti-Irish nativism.

As a homeless and sick immigrant woman with severe gynecological ailments, Smith sought treatment in the charity ward of the newly opened Woman's Hospital of the State of New York in 1855. Her name was the first one listed in the hospital's admittance records.[20] Smith developed her reproductive and gynecological conditions in Ireland. She had first given birth at twenty-one years old, and she described both her labor and delivery as difficult. By the time she immigrated to Manhattan, complications from her earlier delivery had caused Smith to develop the worst case of obstetrical fistula that Dr. Sims had ever seen. While performing a pelvic examination on Smith, Sims and his protégé, Thomas Addis Emmet, noticed a strange mass in her upper vaginal area. The surgeons excised a fishing-net covered wooden ball, used as a pessary, from her scar tissue. The ball, which had been inserted while she lived in Ireland, was used to keep her fallen womb inside her body. Additionally, she had a herniated bladder that had also prolapsed. She had become incontinent, her vulva had been rubbed raw because of urine leakage, and her stench, caused by rectal and vaginal incontinence, made her a "most offensive and loathsome object," according to Sims.[21]

As he had during the mid- to late 1840s with his enslaved experimental patients, Sims operated on Smith numerous times without anesthesia in front of many onlookers. In Smith's case, Sims and Emmet performed thirty surgeries on her over a period of six years. Although Sims left the country in 1859 to perform gynecological surgeries such as clitoridectomies in Europe, his junior colleague, Thomas Emmet, continued to work on Smith until the early 1860s. Over this period of time, Sims operated on Mary Smith even more frequently than he had on his enslaved patients. Additionally, Smith was allowed to work in the hospital performing menial labor just as Sims's enslaved patients worked under his watchful eye in the Alabama fistula-repair hospital he had had built for them.

As a southerner and former slave owner, James Marion Sims, along with his Virginia-born junior colleague, Thomas Emmet, was familiar with surveilling women's bodies, especially those who fell outside the bounds of racial and class normativity.[22] As in Alabama, Sims eventually lost the support of his community at the Woman's Hospital, particularly fellow doctors and board members.

The Woman's Hospital's Board of Directors threatened to dismiss him because of the number of onlookers in the medical theater during operations.[23] It is unclear whether the board threatened Sims with dismissal out of respect for patients, or if it was a case of order for the hospital.

Although Sims was reliving some of the same infamy he had experienced as a doctor to slave women, he did diverge from his usual practices with regard to publications. He did not publish any articles about his surgical work on Mary Smith, even though his early surgical interventions with her were successful. For a doctor who was such a prolific medical writer, it is confounding that Sims did not seek publication on this set of fistula surgeries. Perhaps he remained silent about this case because he had botched his last surgery on Smith's vulva and vagina. Sims had removed bladder stones from her, and in his attempt to do so, he had irreversibly ruined the meticulous surgical work that Emmet had performed on Smith during Sims's residency in Europe. Sims's mistake created another fistula and damaged the tissue surrounding Smith's urethra. He abandoned his treatment of her and left her in almost the same physical shape in which he had initially found her over five years prior. Sadly, she died two years later, as a "common street beggar" not far from the Woman's Hospital.[24]

The staggering numbers of poverty-stricken Irish immigrant women like Mary Smith, who suffered from various physical ailments, helped to create an urban nascent welfare system. One of the thrusts of this kind of northern reform was to provide medical care for the poor, and immigrants overwhelmingly constituted this lot. Historian Kevin Kenny notes that in New York, the majority of Irish-born people lived in the city's poorest wards, the "First, Fourth and Sixth," amid deplorable living conditions. Kenny also found that by the "1850s, as many as 30,000 Irish men, women and children, could be found living in cellars in New York City, without light or drainage." The Irish "accounted for an estimated 70 per cent of the recipients of charity and over 60 per cent of the population of almshouses."[25] As a result, nineteenth-century antebellum-era Irish immigration was markedly different from earlier cycles of European immigration. Irish immigrant women tended to be single and older than previous European women immigrants entering the United States. They were also poorer as a whole; by the 1850s, the Irish made up 51.2 percent of poorhouse populations in Buffalo, New York.[26] Popular newspaper editor Hezekiah Niles, a nativist, wrote a number of articles detailing his disdain for the Irish because they, in his estimation, overcrowded city almshouses and were an economic burden on communities collectively and specifically on native-born white Americans.[27]

Already dealing with racist ideas about themselves as "lustful" and "hyper-sexed" creatures, poor Irish-born women also suffered from a prevailing dogma that they were incapable of exercising self-control. The fact that a disproportionate number of poor Irish immigrant women worked in the sex trade placed many of them in the position of becoming single mothers. Unlike slave women, there was little "worth" attached to Irish women who birthed children as single women. A reporter with the *New York Independent* sarcastically wrote, "Did wealth consist in children, it is well known, that the Irish would be rich people."[28] In an examination of sex and reproduction, Helen Lefkowitz Horowitz writes, "An important motive behind understanding the sexual body in the nineteenth century arose from the drive to control reproduction."[29] Although white Americans were concerned with Irish women's high birthrates, their concerns and consternation did not result in total control of Irish women's reproduction as it did for enslaved women. In the American imagination, Irish women immigrants, like black women, embodied unbridled sexual immorality. Due to the disproportionately high rates of Irish immigrant women who were jailed because of prostitution and the high number of births outside marriage among them, this group of women seemed to perfectly fit the country's idea of the sexually promiscuous and deviant woman.[30] So within this context it is understandable that Hezekiah Niles had such animosity toward the Irish.

Similarly to journalists, medical doctors were also publishing articles that extended the anti-Irish critique to describe the sexual lives and gynecological conditions of Irish women. In these journals, doctors used revealing language that was strikingly similar to speech they employed to detail enslaved black women's bodies and sexual behaviors. In an 1838 article in the *American Journal of Medical Sciences*, Dr. J. B. S. Jackson related a conversation that his colleague, Dr. Ezra Palmer, had with an Irish patient at the House of Industry in South Boston, a poorhouse.[31] The Irish woman was questioned after the death of her German roommate. The patient shared that the twenty-five-year-old German woman intimated to her that she "had a child in her own country." Jackson did not believe the Irish woman's account. He wrote, "As will appear by the dissection, this must have been impossible. . . . She was never married, and . . . she was the daughter of a respectable farmer; the story may have been fabricated by the person who told it, from the love for falsehood which many of the low Irish seem to have."[32] The autopsy later revealed that the German woman was hermaphroditic; she did not have a uterus. The doctor privileged his class biases over the possibility that the daughter of a "respectable farmer" might have lied about motherhood.

These kinds of medical experiences were happening throughout the North. In 1840 Pennsylvania, Dr. George T. Dexter was asked by a colleague to examine an eighteen-year-old Irish girl who suffered from persistent hiccups that caused her to convulse violently.[33] What transpired over the next few months proved so unsettling for the patient that she ran away from her home, the site of her medical treatments. After several visits over a period of about two months, a nurse informed Dexter that the girl had wanted "to cut off a wart on her leg."[34] He soon discovered from the patient that she had several warts, but they were "genital" warts. The teen told the doctor that when she "cut them off the hiccough subsided." She then confided that she had been masturbating for two years to stop the hiccoughs. It was after her confession that Dr. Dexter determined he needed to "test" the veracity of her statements. His assessment included pressing "gently but firmly upon the clitoris outside her linen, with [his] my hand, and the convulsions gradually subsided, and she went to sleep."[35] During the next day's visit the girl informed Dexter that her hiccups were caused this time because she hit her back against her bedpost. Dexter decided that clitoral stimulation would stop her hiccups and spasms. His clitoral-based treatment went on for nearly four months. This was a strange curative practice for a doctor to choose, for he had derived, from his patient's revelations, that masturbation caused her hiccups.

Dexter was allegedly disgusted by the details of the girl's masturbation, although he continued questioning her about the practice. He stated, "She did not seem to have any hesitation in answering my questions." He even added in his notes that the young woman revealed to him, "so great" was her "venereal passion," that she carried to bed with her, a constant companion, a large piece of *wood shaped like a penis*" (italics in the original).[36] As exceptional as this case is, it becomes even stranger. Not wanting to be "deceived," Dexter brought in several of his "professional brethren" to examine and treat the teenager. They found that her hiccups and spasms were caused by spinal pressure, and the cure was genital stimulation. The doctor also believed she was unaware of her "depraved condition" because she was a member of a local religious society that he considered immoral. The course of treatment stopped, not because Dexter and his colleagues ended it but because the girl "left town." He seemed surprised that "she did without informing" him "of her intention to do so."[37]

The fact that George T. Dexter could publish a "Singular Case of Hiccough Caused by Masturbation" in a leading medical journal exemplifies how Irish women's sexual lives, like black women's sexualities, could be discussed indiscriminately, bluntly, and easily. Dexter's Irish immigrant patient experienced a twofold gaze: a metaphorical one from the medical journal's readership and a literal one from the team of doctors assembled to "cure" her of her "venereal passions" and hiccups.[38]

Like the pregnant enslaved woman mentioned in the first chapter whose genitalia were exposed publicly as she lay bleeding on the kitchen floor of her master's house, the treatment of the young Irish woman demonstrates how doctors treated and wrote about black and foreign-born women without thought to their sensibilities. In journal articles, black and Irish women served as flesh-and-blood symbols of biological abnormalities linked to race. This act of framing was a function of the social process of not only defining difference but also identifying how to respond to "otherness." As a medical doctor, Dexter could link disease to socially unacceptable behavior such as masturbation, a "capricious" attitude, and even running away from home secretly. Although he and his peers relied on masturbation to cure this woman, in Dexter's article, only the patient was deemed sexually deviant. However, the tenor of these men's writings reflects their belief that racial difference existed between them and the patient. Also, at the heart of the doctor's anger over his patient's running away from home was his consternation that he could not continue treating her and could only guess the specific causes of her condition and not name it definitively. As medical historian Charles Rosenberg argues, "If it [illness] is not specific, it is not a disease, and a sufferer is not entitled to the sympathy . . . connection with an agreed-upon diagnosis."[39]

Medical journals and the rise of gynecology allowed a new group of professionally trained doctors legitimate spaces to introduce and strengthen their racialized attitudes concerning the medical lives of racially stigmatized people and their supposed pathologies. Specifically during the antebellum era, an emergent class of gynecologists and other doctors integrated science and biology as they framed and defined diseases, gynecological ones included. Through their medical practices and professional writings, they began to define medicine. Medical educator Alan Gregg describes these men's work as "the study and application of biology in a matrix that is at once historical, social, political, economic, and cultural."[40]

As scientific racism became bio-racism, many early American gynecologists were participating in creating theories about race and gender, especially about black and white women although they knew that these women's physical bodies were intrinsically the same. Bio-racism integrated both medical and scientific research to prove how biologically distinct black and white people were from each other. Antebellum-era white supremacy did not allow a space for one to address this kind of racialized cognitive dissonance. For example, Charles Meigs, a noted Philadelphia gynecologist, shared with his students the following assessment of women via his published lectures. He stated that a woman was "a moral, a sexual, a germiferous, gestative and parturient creature."[41] Although he did not describe women racially, the racial climate and etiquette of the day dictated that he was referring to the white woman as the universal representative model for all women. Yet it was the preserved womb of a black cancer victim that Meigs displayed in his Philadelphia museum as a teaching tool for his colleagues to learn how cancer affected all women's uteri. The universal template for woman might have been white, but the fluidity of nineteenth-century racial categories could expand to include whoever fit a doctor's medical needs at any given time.

Pioneering gynecologists like Meigs knew the importance of medical writings within society. Their publications helped their peers understand the varied medical experiences of Irish women. Historian Alan Kraut has reported how doctors compared Irish immigrant women patients to other European immigrant women. One doctor wrote, "Germans were praised [because] . . . they seemed 'docile and affectionate' to the doctors . . . the reverse was said of the Irish." Another doctor described a mentally ill Irish patient as having "nymphomania," and he linked the disorder to her morality. He described her as "vulgar," just as Dr. Dexter characterized his Irish teenage patient as immoral.[42] Clearly, the public nature of these women's sexual behaviors made them easy targets for doctors to moralize against them. Medical men also knew that these women were not "normal" by nineteenth-century definitions, and yet these women were further penalized for their Irishness.

These medical journal articles also inform scholars about how indigent Irish-born women made decisions about their bodies and responded to medical procedures they underwent as a result of lengthy hospital stays. In 1844, C.C., a nineteen-year-old pregnant woman, was admitted to the Philadelphia Almshouse and Hospital to deliver her child. Dr. George Burnwell, the physician who treated her, described C.C. using three adjectives, "short, stout Irish."[43] Arguably, Burnwell used a lexicon that linked race and class and inferred that despite the obstetrical problems that the pregnant teenager might have had, as an Irish woman, she was strong and healthy. C.C. represented a flesh-and-blood metonym for the urban white scourge: she was a poor, unmarried Irish woman who relied on charity during her pregnancy and childbirth.

Nineteen hours passed, and C.C. had still not given birth. Alarmed, doctors bled the young woman and administered ergot, a rye-based pharmaceutical that was used to induce uterine contractions during deliveries. After two days, Dr. Burnwell knew that C.C. would deliver a stillborn baby; he had to surgically remove her fetus. Immediately after he began the procedure, the young woman's "uterus fell away," and doctors administered stimulants to revive her.[44] She entered the hospital to give birth and left the building childless and sterile.

Like C.C., Irish immigrant women created and responded to the interventions made into their medical lives in various ways. Some obtained professional medical help, some entered the field of nursing, some relied on home-based traditional medicines, and some sought solace away from the formal medical gaze of white men. It is important to understand this group of women within the context of a comparative medical model that highlights how modern American gynecology impacted their lives. Historians of the antebellum era have drawn comparisons between the oppression of enslaved people of African descent and that of poor Irish immigrants for several generations in their scholarship on whiteness, race, politics, and identity. This scholarship has centered on the development of black and Irish nationalism, the political economy of slavery, and the wage slavery that recently immigrated Irish laborers suffered under during the nineteenth century. Yet the medical lives and experiences of Irish immigrant women were not parsed for careful analytic review.

Labor relations were sometimes present in boss-doctor-patient exchanges. It was a common practice that employers intervened on behalf of their domestic servants if the women were exceedingly ill. During the mid-1860s, Mary McC.'s boss sent the twenty-one-year-old Irish cook to be examined by leading gynecologist Dr. T. Gaillard Thomas at either Bellevue or Charity Hospital in New York City.[45] How could Mary McC. decline the services of Dr. Thomas if she had no initial say in selecting him as her physician? Young Irish immigrants did not have a long American culture of traditional and naturalistic health care as did enslaved women. Clearly, when writing about the ethical policies that governed doctor-patient relationships, the AMA conveniently imagined patients as either white men or white women. The poor and immigrants who were relegated to tenement living seemed not to be considered by doctors; they lay outside the power structure where medical men could only negotiate and barter power with white men and perhaps elite white women.

The starkest difference that existed in the treatment of these enslaved black women and Irish immigrant women lay in what happened to them after their surgical encounters. As their sick bodies were healed, black women returned to slave communities to toil. Poor Irish women's improved health status allowed them to continue to work for wages as free women. Thus, the development of the domestic service industry in northeastern cities like New York and Boston has a direct link to the work of early gynecologists. These men were responsible for "fixing" Bridget's body ("Bridget" was a derisive name for Irish women).

Irish women who married and gave birth to children were afforded opportunities to improve their lots in life because they were not owned, no matter the dire circumstances they faced. They did so by vending, educating their children, and marrying native-born American white men. Many second-generation Irish women became nurses and teachers because of the efforts of their mothers. Further, the American-born daughters of Irish immigrant women did not face the risks of sexual abuse that occurred aboard ships sailing from Ireland to America. This situation also heightened the differences between the daughters of poor immigrants and enslaved women. Enslaved girls would always be subject to the same abuse that their mothers had suffered and could not rely on education to better their situation. Although many Irish immigrant servants, like their enslaved sisters in the South, were at the mercy of sometimes-unscrupulous employers who took advantage of them sexually, the fact remained that Irish immigrant women could choose to leave their employers. Throughout northern cities, the number of Catholic-run charitable organizations located in Irish tenements directly dealt with issues of sexual abuse. Slave women did not have the same kind of formal mechanisms in place to deal with complex and damaging issues like rape and molestation by their owners.

Irish immigrant women also relied on the Catholic Church to be involved in their healing. The reality for this group of women was that, unlike enslaved women, they could integrate their religious beliefs into the formalized hospitals they used. Irish Catholic sisters and the subsequent charitable organizations that they ran created "cultural sites" for healing to occur. To combat nativists' beliefs that the Irish would be "a permanent dependent class in America," these Irish-Catholic spaces proved that Irish-born women could be enterprising, productive, and "clean" citizens.[46]

Sick women who battled gynecological illnesses or who had complicated pregnancies were often at the receiving end of doctors' maltreatment. Mary Donovan, a pregnant woman with a spinal deformity, was one of those whom Dr. George Elliot, a Bellevue Hospital physician, recognized as needing his medical assistance. Elliot treated her in March 1857 and published a medical article about her birthing process with language bloated with descriptors that demeaned her body, intellect, class, and ultimately her race. While the doctor might have simply written clinical notes in dry and apolitical technical language, Elliot's records of Donovan's case demonstrate just how pervasive nineteenth-century ideas about biological differences were in women's medicine.

Elliot first wrote his patient's name, Mary Donovan, and the second word he used to describe her was "Irish." He observed that the thirty-year-old first-time mother "attracted [his] observation . . . by her deformity." After querying Mary for a few minutes about her pregnancy and her spinal deformity, Elliot determined she was a woman who possessed a "very low order of intelligence" and was "apt to exaggerate." Elliot wrote that most of the pregnant women in the charity lying-in ward, where Donovan was hospitalized, lied about the dates they had become pregnant so that they could keep receiving "charity."[47]

After Donovan was informed that she would probably endure a difficult delivery, she gave Elliot her consent to quicken her delivery by administering a warm-water douche to induce labor. The doctor initially wanted to administer carbolic acid gas but decided against it due to time constraints. (Doctors in the 1850s used carbolic acid gas for the "treatment of painful affections of the uterus" and to "induce artificial *accouchement*" or labor.)[48] Once the treatment began, Donovan offered "insane struggles" to stop the douching. She fought so vigorously to release herself from the restraints of the medical staff that Elliot finally administered chloroform to calm her.[49] After two days of the douche treatment, Donovan delivered a son on March 23, 1857, but he died a few hours later.[50] During Donovan's treatment, four other doctors observed her along with Elliot. Her case was later used as a pedagogical tool in the pages of *New York Medical Journal* so that other physicians could learn how to perfect his douching method on other pregnant women. Elliot described Donovan as a patient who was violent, dumb, and defective, but her body provided a pathway for doctors to learn more about all laboring bodies even though she lost her baby in the process of his treatment.

Some Irish immigrant women acted outside gendered ideals and possessed physical abnormalities that encouraged doctors like Elliot to use women such as Mary Donovan to establish a race-and-religion-specific matrix that exceptionalized poor Irish-born women. Descriptions of Irish immigrant women in the medical literature are remarkably similar to the way doctors wrote about enslaved women's bodies; black women were either amazingly strong or weakened when "white" blood was apparent. The *Georgia Blister and Critic*, an antebellum-era medical journal, published an excerpt of *Types of Mankind*, a book about mulatto women authored by controversial physicians Josiah Nott and George Gliddon. The article illustrates how some physicians used their writings to promote scientific ideas about biological distinctiveness. Nott and Gliddon wrote "that the *mulatto women* are peculiarly delicate, and subject to a variety of chronic diseases. That they are bad breeders, bad nurses, liable to abortions, and that their children generally die young."[51] One Irish physician wrote about the so-called peculiarities of pregnant Irish women in the *Boston Medical and Surgical Journal*. He urged doctors to rely on the traditional practice of bloodletting on pregnant Irish women because of "the strong, almost insurmountable obstinacy of the Irish with us."[52]

Some Irish immigrant women were like Eliza B., a thirty-five-year-old Irish nanny who suffered from gynecological ailments but resisted the absolute authority of medical doctors.[53] Eliza, who was single, suffered from the pain of an enlarged ovarian cyst for eighteen months. Her attending physician, Dr. T. Gaillard Thomas, one of the country's leading gynecologists, initially described her as possessing a "morbid disposition." The first physicians she saw misdiagnosed her as being pregnant. Eliza B. lived with severe abdominal pain for two years. Perhaps her "morbid disposition" arose from the fact that doctors initially dismissed her pain. She finally checked into a hospital on November 1, 1862, and agreed to undergo an ovariotomy.[54]

The medical case of Mrs. F., a thirty-five-year-old mother of three who lived in Philadelphia, demonstrates how Irish immigrant women relied on each other and asserted their autonomy in obstetrical and gynecological cases.[55] Apparently very busy, Mrs. F. experienced a violent fall as she held her "quite heavy" infant while she attempted to use her chamber pot.[56] Unfortunately, she was well into her fourth pregnancy. Dr. Gegan visited her on the morning of January 30, 1859, to examine her. She had lain on her right side for twelve hours because she was in such immense pain, was weak, and was vomiting. During his visit, he determined that she must have ruptured her uterus even though he "could not reach the os uteri [cervix opening]."[57]

At one o' clock the next afternoon, Gegan asked if Mrs. F. believed that her child was alive. She stated, "I feel it all the time."[58] After the physician left, she called her circle of women friends to nurse her during his absence and also to provide community care during her medical crisis. Trusting her five friends to safely change her position in the bed, Mrs. F. asked her them to physically turn her body on her left side. Upon Dr. Gegan's arrival that night, she hastily offered an excuse for why her friends were lifting her; she allegedly felt "much better" and no longer suffered from "soreness on the right side."[59] A few hours before her death, Mrs. F told the doctor that "she could distinctly feel the child move."[60] Shortly after 7:30 P.M. on January 31, 1859, Mrs. F. died.

Dr. Gegan noted that the late patient's husband was quite moved by his wife's statement. The doctor remarked that Mr. F. agreed, only after his wife's death, "that I should attempt the removal of the child, by abdominal incision."[61] Dr. Gegan respected the husband's wishes regarding the performance of an autopsy. The politics of nineteenth-century respectability were being performed fully. Women were almost always seen as meddlesome when involved in male affairs, yet the doctor allowed "four or five" of Mrs. F.'s women friends to comfort her even while he was present. The doctor treated his Irish patient as a white "lady" for reasons he did not disclose, but one can assume she was accorded respect because she was married and perhaps so desperately wanted her child to live.

In another obstetrical case involving an Irish immigrant obstetrical patient, surgeons at the Philadelphia Hospital aided "Alice Mailey during her delivery." In 1859, Mailey was placed under the care of nurses and physicians at the Nurse's Home.[62] She was twenty-nine years old, unmarried, primiparous, and considered healthy. Like the pregnancies of many women of the time, however, Mailey's became complicated. She was placed under the care of Dr. D. Hayes Agnew, one of the nation's leading surgeons. In a medical journal article, Agnew described Mailey's childbirth as "severe."[63] During her protracted delivery, her uterus "ruptured," and the fetus shifted "into the abdomen."[64] The baby was delivered stillborn, and the mother was left with a "rent in the uterine walls" that had "extended through the cervix, and involved the vesico-vaginal fistula septum, giving rise to a fistula [hole]."[65] Agnew operated on Mailey four times, first at the Nurse's Home and later at Saint Joseph's Hospital, for the repair of her vesico-vaginal fistula.[66] After Mailey's recovery, Agnew reported that she not only "enjoyed comfortable health" but also was "able to support herself as a servant in a private family."[67]

These immigrant women's medical experiences show the range of treatment that Irish women received from doctors, from sympathetic to bigoted, and highlight some of the differences between their situations and that of enslaved women. Whiteness was extended to Alice Mailey, Eliza B., and Mrs. F., an act that no enslaved woman was ever given in the antebellum era.

By the early 1860s, as political definitions of blackness and whiteness were becoming firmer, native-born white Americans began to slowly extend a few privileges of whiteness to Irish women. However, early gynecologists were still writing about their bodies as if they were more "colored" than white. As Americans continued to cultivate their brand of nationalism, medicine and medical writings served as sites where race was being reified. After the Civil War, legislators in the former Confederate states created Black Codes, laws that used language from scientific racism to distinguish black people, white people, and "mulattos" from each other. Gynecologists who wrote about biological differences helped to create the environment from which those racist laws sprang. In their writings, they proclaimed that elite, native-born white women were fragile, normal women. Irish and black women, in contrast, were described as physically stronger and more sexual, and they were believed to suffer reproductive ailments at different rates than white women did. It was a nearly universal belief that black women and Irish women were more fertile than their white counterparts. Early gynecologists continued to promote the idea that these women were apelike and "more suitable" for gynecological experiments than white women.[68] Historian Laura Briggs has noted the contradictions in early gynecologists' writings about immigrant women and black women, who were supposed to have easier childbirths. Early gynecologists' writings featured Irish women who had protracted labors that lasted for days and were so difficult that medical men were involved, an unusual practice during the nineteenth century.[69] Often Irish women were mentioned in articles about the effects of multiple births. Dr. William Potts Dewees, one of the country's most prominent obstetricians, saw one married Irish woman, Mrs. Haley, in July 1830 and detailed her fecundity and gynecological conditions. Haley was sixty years old, the mother of sixteen children, and apparently was still suffering from her many pregnancies. Potts Dewees wrote that his patients had "suffer[ed] 3 abortions, early labour . . . she ha[d] suffered with the present prolapsus the past 6 years."[70] Regardless of the contradictions they contained, medical writings about immigrant and black women represented one of the most popular sites for ideologies about black and white biological distinctions to be introduced and discussed.

Medical doctors and scientists who researched biological differences among the "races" connected Irish women to black women for reasons ranging from their supposed superior physical strength to their fecundity. By the end of the nineteenth century, physicians like Lucien Warner were thoroughly convinced that black and Irish women shared the same reproductive capabilities and superior health. Warner posited, "The African negress, who toils beside her husband in the fields of the south, and Bridget who washes, and scrubs, and toils in our homes at the north, enjoy for the most part good health, with comparative immunity from uterine diseases."[71]

Gynecologists' construction of black and immigrant women's reproductive bodies as "medical superbodies" was a means to make sense of these women medically and also a rationale for how they were to be treated outside medical spaces. As noted in an earlier chapter, James Marion Sims's father expressed disappointment with his son's decision to pursue medicine. He believed there was no science, respect, or honor in the field. So for men like Sims who were as committed to healing patients as they were to establishing respectable, honorable, and lucrative careers, more than medical knowledge was at stake. They were contributing to the greater good by using bodies that were "fit for labor" to heal all bodies. Black lives mattered medically because they made white lives healthier and better. It was important for journal readers to know how these women, the unrecognized and often unnamed "mothers of gynecology," responded to examinations, surgeries, experimentations, and even recovery because this knowledge enabled white men to more easily grasp science-based theories that explained why blackness, and to a lesser degree, Irishness, was so strange and pathological. The addition of disenfranchised Irish immigrant women to biomedical explorations of racial otherness did not explode existing categories but rather continued discussions about these women as one-dimensional objects to be understood without nuance. The medical narratives that were created based on these women's gynecological treatment helped to further perpetuate the uneven cultural productions on biologically based racial difference. Racial categories were still being processed in the antebellum era, but modern American gynecology's growth worked to lay a foundation on which both blackness and whiteness would be defined as separate and unequal for generations. The black female body was central to these discussions and medical knowledge productions.

·❬═══════════════════❭·

CHAPTER FIVE

HISTORICAL BLACK SUPERBODIES
AND THE MEDICAL GAZE

They bear surgical operations much better than white
people; and what would be the cause of insupportable pain
to a white man, a negro would almost disregard.

—Dr. Charles White

Negroes, on the other hand it is well known, are negligent
of themselves, especially when, from the nature of the
case, the treatment has to be long continued.

—Henry F. and Robert Campbell,
founders of Jackson Street Hospital and Surgical
Infirmary for Negroes in Augusta, Georgia

INVOKING THE MEMORY OF DR. JAMES MARION SIMS'S SLAVE PATIENTS
and the advancement of modern American gynecology at Sims's November
1883 funeral, leading obstetrician Dr. William Waring Johnston stated in his
eulogy, "Who can tell how many more years the progress of the art might
have been delayed, if the humble negro servitors had not brought their willing sufferings and patient endurance" to assist Dr. Sims's research.[1] Contrary
to Johnston's assertion, however, these sick black women, representing both
Sims's slave patients and his nurses, were experimented and operated on because their masters permitted them to be, not because of their autonomy. Informed consent did not exist for slave patients. They could bring neither their
"sufferings" nor "patient endurance" to the "Father of Gynecology" as free

agents. Dr. Johnston praised Sims's enslaved gynecological patients because the late doctor was being lauded as not only a pioneering medical doctor in the field of women's medicine but also as the sort of slave master whom black women would obey willingly. In Johnston's pronouncement about gynecology's advancement, black women's bodies were normalized, even if for a brief moment, because they were made so by a white man, even before their surgeries. As a son of the South, Johnston could invoke and easily remember docile slave servants happy and willing to give their bodies over for medical research.

This chapter refines the concept of "medical superbodies," which is not a nineteenth-century term but one that describes the myriad ways in which white society and medical men thought of, wrote about, and treated black women in bondage. White medical men tended to write and speak about enslaved black women's bodies, their fecundity, their alleged hypersexuality, and their physical strength, which was supposedly superior to that of white women. At the same time, white doctors rarely attributed qualities that were seen as natural to white women to black women. These men did not map traits such as beauty, humility, patience, and meekness onto black women in slavery. As medical superbodies, sick black women were expected to still perform the duties fit for slaves such as intense agricultural labor and domestic work even while pregnant, infirm, or recovering from illness. It is ironic that black women could be thought of in this white supremacist culture as both physically inferior and superior. The term "medical superbodies" helps clarify how these unintentional gynecological contributions of these women fit into past dialectics surrounding issues of biology, race, normalcy, and medicine. Novelist Toni Morrison, writing about oppression, gender, and black womanhood, opined that to understand these concepts, they must be "situated in the miasma of black life."[2] Slavery produced miasmas that polluted all within its reach, including doctors who brought their racial prejudices into examination rooms. It was out of this already putrid environment that the black medical superbody was birthed and came to represent a being that was treated as something between human and lower primate in sickness and in health.

As early as the 1700s, European scientists were deeply involved in the work of trying to define race and rank human beings according to wide-ranging factors that took into account climate, hue, and a host of other reasons. "During the eighteenth century," as medical humanities scholar Andrew Curran has argued, "the concept of blackness was increasingly dissected, handled, measured, weighed, and used as a demonstrable wedge between human categories."[3] French scientist Georges Cuvier's "explicit instructions on how to procure human skeletons" paints a picture of how racial bigotry infused the work of leading European researchers of the period. Theorist Anne Fausto-

Sterling states that Cuvier informed travelers who visited distant and "exotic" lands to "nab bodies whenever they observed a battle involving 'savages.' "[4] Scientists began to integrate women into their work as they examined and categorized "savage races" that they believed to be inferior. In a glaring example of racial chauvinism, early naturalist Johann Blumenbach presented his ideas about why African babies possessed broad noses and full lips, which he considered unsightly. Blumenbach believed that black mothers' carelessness while breastfeeding and performing agricultural labor caused babies faces to be smashed and consequently, their features were flattened.[5] By the nineteenth century, anthropologists, doctors, and scientists' research about women had morphed into both race science and American gynecology.

As a field, gynecology seemed well suited to perform acts of "racecraft," a term that scholars Barbara and Karen Fields coined as "shorthand" for the process that "transforms *racism*, something an aggressor does, into race, something the target is." Medical men could then conduct an "ultimately vain search for traits with which to demarcate human groups" through their observations and research. They could disseminate their biology-based findings and theories in their medical writings.[6] In a not-so-surprising twist, the normal/abnormal binary that doctors relied on to create newer ideas about racial superiority and inferiority often inverted the era's reigning medical paradigm. Black people and their blackness, seen as a debilitating medical condition, could also serve as a marker for how to make white people better when they fell ill. The medical writings of these physicians laid bare "the role of race as a metalanguage, a theoretical device linking race, class, and gender," and brought attention to its "powerful, all-encompassing effect of the construction and representation of other social and power relations, namely, gender, class, and sexuality."[7]

As doctors, scientists, legislators, and intellectuals reified ideas about racial difference, antebellum-era gynecology provided another platform where abstractions about black people and blackness could become concrete and gain more legitimacy. The antebellum thinkers were simply continuing the work left for them by their intellectual forefathers. Eighteenth-century anthropologists and anatomists formed these types of ideologies because they believed that "African women's alleged extraordinary ease in parturition seemed to indicate pelvises more capacious than European women's . . . (this was also assumed to be true of apes and other quadrupeds)."[8] In 1828 a white plantation overseer in South Carolina felt comfortable and confident enough to borrow medical language and share his observations in a slave management journal about pregnant slave women's deliveries although he was not a medical doctor. He wrote that bondwomen's child-birthing sessions were "reduced one half" in comparison to white women.[9] It seemed that white men's ideas about black women's reproduction proved foundational for accepting broader and more damaging ideas about black people generally. If black women recovered from childbirth more quickly, experienced surgeries without pain, and had oversized genitalia, perhaps America was right to keep the entire "race" enslaved. It is no wonder that the famed antebellum-era physician Samuel Cartwright was asked by his medical colleagues in Louisiana to author an article that would provide scientific evidence about the "Diseases and Peculiarities of the Negro Race."[10] For all the articles published, scientific and medical theories introduced, and laws adopted that affirmed the biological differences between black and white people, the results from medical experimentation should have been the biggest obstacle to racist claims—but they were not.

Gynecological experimentation relied on the sick bodies of women of color and poor women who were considered not quite white to heal white women. Experimentation should have brought into question the very premise of biological differences between black and white people. Doctors should have broken with the shibboleths of racial science because they were examining, treating, and ultimately curing black and white women using identical surgeries. Their work confirmed that it would have been fruitless to employ wholly different surgical techniques on bodies that needed to be not only repaired but also kept alive after these procedures. The magnitude of their deeply held racist ideologies, however, was enough to obscure the findings of these medical men that black and white bodies were anatomically the same.

The following case about Dr. Sims's first enslaved fistula patient elucidates this point in greater detail. In May 1845, eighteen-year-old Lucy of Macon County, Alabama, had recently given birth, during which she experienced deep vaginal ripping. After two months had passed, the severity of her injury prompted her owner, Tom Zimmerman, to send her to Dr. Sims, who lived some miles away, for treatment.[11] After Sims diagnosed Lucy as incurable, he stated that she was "very much disappointed." She stayed at Sims's slave farm a few days before returning to her owner, where she remained until Sims persuaded her owner that he could repair her obstetrical fistula through experimental medical intervention.[12] During Lucy's initial stay over, Sims examined two other enslaved patients suffering from vesico-vaginal fistulae, Anarcha and Betsy, and became convinced that he could also repair their fistulae. Lucy, Anarcha, and Betsy had no clue that their owners would eventually lease them to Sims for five years. Slavery was an institution predicated on migration and control, but one imagines that these young women did not know that their surgeries would be public events for local white townsfolk, that their bodies would be operated on experimentally. They certainly could not have known that over a century later, they would emerge as potent medical symbols of slavery's role in American gynecology's development.

Dr. Sims contacted "about a dozen doctors . . . to witness the series of [fistulae] experiments" he would undertake for five years. Naked, Lucy climbed onto the operation table, got on her knees while two white male medical assistants restrained her. Sims would name this posture "the Sims Position." The illustration of Sims working on one of his experimental fistula patients (fig. 5.1) reveals much about race, respectability, and gynecology. Sims never denied his work on enslaved women, but in an image published about his pioneering work, he is pictured with a white woman nurse and a fully clad white woman patient who is even allowed to keep on her shoes. The illustration, drawn some years after his experimentation ended and meant to recapture that historical moment, whitewashes his use of the Alabama slaves as experimental subjects and nurses. In the image, Sims seems to be guiding his nurse to use the speculum on the white patient. He has his right hand on the patient's thigh to gently keep her vagina open enough for the nurse to maneuver and the medical staff to observe the procedure. His left hand rests on the upper corner of the patient's right buttock. He and the patient appear passive while the white nurse does the indelicate work of inserting the speculum and touching the patient's genitals. This imagined scene portrays white fistula patients as docile, gentle, and soft. It is a fiction that visually effaced the bodies and real experiences of women who had to absorb pain so much that Sims would write of Lucy as someone "bore the operation with great heroism and bravery."[13] In his autobiography, Sims noted that Lucy's bladder had become inflamed postsurgery and her "agony was extreme."[14] Yet medical men like Sims and years later his eulogizer, Dr. Johnston, chose to obfuscate her pain and highlight Lucy's medical role as "a humble negro servitor."

Although Dr. Charles White, whose remark on black and white people's differing sensitivity to pain opens this chapter, believed that black people could tolerate surgery with disregard to pain, Dr. Sims's description of Lucy's "agony," a degree of suffering that exceeds pain, reveals the falsity of White's belief. Sims held fast to the practice of restraining surgical patients because he knew so many of them would physically resist being cut by his surgeon's blade, even black women who were allegedly impervious to surgical pain. The hypocrisy of medical and scientific racism allowed doctors to write about black women's supposed bravery and silence in the face of life-threatening and painful operations while also describing how they were restrained physically. The reality is that medical men, based on their experiences with black patients, did not believe that black people did not experience any pain. Instead, they believed

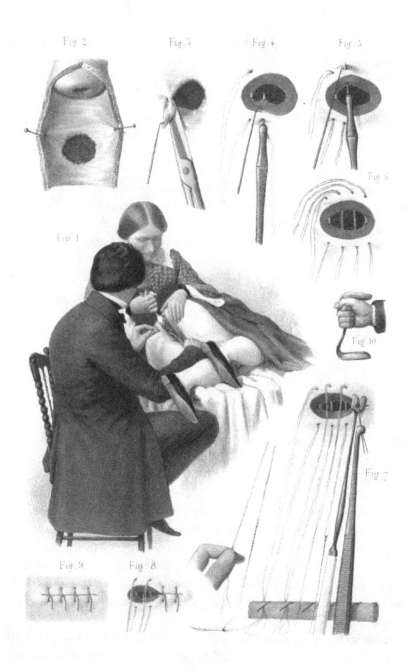

FIGURE 5.1. Dr. James Marion Sims and nurse
repairing a vesico-vaginal fistula patient.

From Henry Savage, *The Surgery, Surgical Pathology,
and Surgical Anatomy of the Female Pelvic Organs,
in a Series of Coloured Plates Taken from Nature*
(London: John Churchill & Sons, 1862).

black people experienced pain that was not as severe as white people's pain. In their writings, nonetheless, they nullified black people's sufferings as a part of the human experience.

Lucy and the other enslaved patients she lived with came to embody either the proper function or the dysfunction of women's reproductive health in doctors' medical writings. Historian Jennifer Morgan has called black women slaves "laboring women" because of the physical and reproductive work they performed across the entire landscape of slavery. The psychological stressors such as fear, depression, and feelings of isolation that laboring women faced as sick slaves, particularly fistula patients who were sometimes forced to live away from other slaves because of their stench, must have impacted them negatively. Added to this collection of psychological symptoms, "laboring women" who were considered medical superbodies came to represent more than the physical and reproductive labor they performed, especially as American gynecological medicine developed alongside racism. For these women, as representative black bodies, the meaning assigned to them held as much meaning as the humiliation, brutality, and violence inflicted on them as white doctors sought knowledge on their bodies.[15] In the case of Lucy and her slave cohorts, Sims trained them to work as his surgical nurses while still serving as subjects of his experimental surgeries after the white community stopped supporting his research.[16] The universe of antebellum-era slavery and gynecological medicine was capacious and malleable enough to provide a space for a slave-owning surgeon to medically train his slave experimental patients so that they, who were deemed intellectually inferior beings because of their race and sex, could help him pioneer a surgical path for healing.

There was a voluminous outpouring of medical texts on the so-called differences between blacks, whites, Celts, and the English, who were thought of as "true" whites. By the mid-1850s, some researchers had concluded that certain "degraded" persons were little more than advanced animals. In his 1852 edition of *Comparative Physiognomy; or, Resemblances between Men and Animals*, early scientist James W. Redfield likened "Negroes to elephants and fish."[17] Redfield also believed that "the noisy Irish immigrant in America . . . was more like 'a scavenger-dog of the city.'"[18]

Scientists and laypersons alike projected a simianized image on people of African descent and the Irish. By the first half of the nineteenth century, scientists had linked certain human beings to apes for well over a century. In the antebellum era, the corresponding images of blacks and Celts as closely related to apes began to materialize in diverse ways that worked in tandem with the racism of the age. In *White over Black*, historian of racial attitudes and slavery Winthrop Jordan documents these early beliefs. Jordan discusses the early attitudes among various Europeans who believed black women to be the sexual partners of apes. He notes, "The notion had scientific value: it forged a crucial link in the Chain of Being and helped explain the Negro's and the ape's prognathism. . . . The sexual union of apes and Negroes was *always* conceived as involving *female Negroes* and *male apes*! Apes had intercourse with Negro *women*."[19]

The nineteenth century was a period in American medicine when doctors were bent on discovering the secrets of the "female animal" in order to both tame and remedy her peculiarities. Antebellum medical convention declared women to be the more delicate sex because of their "finer" and "more irritable" nervous systems.[20] By 1868, some gynecologists had begun to "cure" elite white women of nervousness or "neurasthenia," a condition that allegedly weakened one's nerves, and they did so through clitoridectomies, the removal of their clitorises. This surgery was a manifestation of the chilling belief that nerves and uteri ruled women's behavior. For upper-class white women, who were already burdened with the notion of their biological fragility, white male doctors felt obligated to cure them of any ill that might aggravate their sensitive natures. Clearly, this surgery would not have been performed on black women, enslaved or free, for the same reasons because white doctors perceived black women as not having pathologies related to sensitivity. As historians of medicine Carroll Smith-Rosenberg and Charles Rosenberg articulate in their article "The Female Animal," nineteenth-century medicine definitively declared that substantive emotional differences existed between white men and women.[21] Even leading American gynecologist Charles Meigs proclaimed, "Women possess a peculiar trait—it is modesty. . . . The attribute of modesty . . . binds her to the domestic altar."[22]

Modesty was neither a trait nor a trope that enslaved and poor Irish immigrant women could claim and rely on in their interactions with white male physicians. As such, white medical men claimed that these women were unabashedly explicit in succumbing to their so-called naturally carnal natures, a racist belief that nineteenth-century medical research advanced. Moreover, the Western world seemed to be utterly intrigued with the supposed unbridled sexuality of the poor. The Irish-born were included within these beliefs. The conviction that these women's bodies were somehow "super" in their abilities to transcend pain shaped early gynecologists' behavior toward them on operating tables and in examination rooms.

The scientific and medical beliefs that doctors held about Irish women were nearly indistinguishable to those they held about African women. Historian of gender and science Londa Schiebinger notes in her work on women's roles in the creation of science that pioneering German scientist Johann Blumenbach promoted theories about racial difference in various groups of women.[23] She writes, "Blumenbach . . . argued further that breast size is not a uniform racial characteristic."[24] As a testament to his relatively liberal attitudes about race, he further asserted, that not "all Europeans have small comely breasts" (he mentioned the large breasts of Irish women).[25] By the nineteenth century, the idea of racially marked women such as the Irish and those of African descent was reflected in the specific ways that doctors wrote about them. For example, Dr. Thomas Gallaher of Pennsylvania described his patient "Mrs. F." as a "hearty, robust, and healthy Irish woman" in an 1851 medical journal article about her ruptured uterus.[26] Typically, doctors did not highlight the racial characteristics of patients they considered normal or like themselves.

Although the institutions of women's medicine such as journals and professional organizations outlined how doctors were to treat patients, when race entered the picture, some doctors abandoned the guidelines that they were to follow, as the case of Sims's patient Mary Smith illustrates. The "Code of Ethics" adopted by the AMA dictated that doctors were not to abandon patients: "A physician ought not to abandon a patient because the case is deemed incurable."[27] In James Marion Sims's treatment of his Irish-born patient Mary Smith, Thomas Addis Emmet, his assistant, explicitly stated that Sims abandoned Smith after he botched her final surgery. Article II of the Code of Ethics also highlights the rights of patients. It states, "Patients should prefer a physician whose habits of life are regular," and in cases of the dismissal of a doctor, the patient should utilize "justice and common courtesy" and provide reasons why the dismissal occurred.[28] The limitations of class, however, precluded poor Irish immigrant women, who were treated in police stations, almshouses, jails, and charity hospitals, from being fully able to rely on all the protections granted by the AMA. The status of the medical superbody was applied to women like Mary Smith, whose reproductive bodies failed the doctors that were expected to heal them.

The status of medical superbody was also ascribed to southern white women who violated the racial norms of the slave-holding region. John Archer, the nineteenth-century Maryland physician and surgeon mentioned in chapter 1, made the erroneous race-based claim that black and white women who willfully engaged in consensual sexual relations with men of the opposite race would produce black and mulatto twin children depending on the mother's race. He is credited as citing the country's first documented case of heteropaternal superfecundation, the condition in which two different males impregnate a woman and thereby father fraternal twins. In his article, Archer was clear in his message that both the women and the men in these cases acted outside the parameters of normalcy. His article "Facts Illustrating a Disease Peculiar to the Female Children of Negro Slaves: and Observations, Showing that a White Woman by Intercourse with a White Man and a Negro, May Conceive Twins,

One of Which Shall be White, and the Other a Mulatto; and that, Vice Versa, a Black Woman by Intercourse with a Negro and a White Man, May Conceive Twins, One of Which Shall be a Negro and the Other a Mulatto" highlight two exceptional medical cases that illustrate the multifaceted nature of American racial ideologies. Most telling, the black woman profiled in his article was the only mother capable of birthing a black baby despite being impregnated by a white man. Unlike the white mother of twins, Archer's slave patient seemed unable to produce a white child—although in reality black slave women often birthed white-skinned babies for white men during slavery's long presence in America.

Even more surprisingly, in the same article Archer cited a second example of a black-white union that seemed to prove his claims. He stated, "A white man cohabited with a negro woman after her husband, and the negro woman brought a black child and a mulatto at birth."[29] For Archer, the black female superbody became an "outlawed body."[30] Archer explicitly stated in his journal article that he presented these cases to serve a rather high-minded purpose: he wanted their dissemination to provide an accurate "account" of the "propagation of the human species."[31] Yet Archer chose to focus on miscegenation between black and white people. As an extremely elite Marylander—he was the first person to receive a medical degree in the United States—John Archer was fully aware that sexual relations between black and white people were considered not only taboo but also illegal.[32] His medical case narratives also served as warnings about the dire consequences that existed for black and white people who crossed racial lines sexually. Subsequently, Archer's obstetric patients symbolized superbodies, ones that could birth "marked" babies whose hues represented the stain of either the white or the black female parent who had transgressed sexually.[33]

Applying the concept of the black medical superbody allows for a more nuanced way to examine and understand bonded women's bodies, for every reproductive, gynecologic, and sexual act experienced by them had multiple meanings. For example, the testimony of Hilliard Yellerday, a former slave, reveals the belief that there was little, if any, distinction between slave girls and adult slave women regarding sexual behavior. For slave girls and women, age, childhood, and adulthood were subjective and often arbitrary concepts based on the whims of slave owners or lawmakers. "A slave girl," Yellerday said, "was expected to have children as soon as she became a woman. Some of them had children at the age of twelve and thirteen years old. Negro men six feet tall went to some of these children."[34]

Like their more mature female slave cohorts, older teenaged girls who lived under bondage were also expected to produce children at accelerated rates like "experienced" breeders once they were partnered with slave men. Not only were some enslaved pubescent girls forced to engage in sexual relationships with men, but black women and girls were also required to bear many children like other chattel (cattle, hogs, and chickens) on slave farms and plantations. Nineteenth-century whites embraced the axiom that black women gave birth frequently and easily. While some formerly enslaved persons recalled their mothers bearing as many as twenty children, a few also described the severe and unrealistic notions that masters held about black women's labor and recovery time.[35] Formerly enslaved Ophelia Whitley remembered that in rare instances, her master would force parturient women to "go ter de house an' find a baby an' be back at wuck de next day."[36] Yet the concerns about their enslaved women breeding that some slaveholders and doctors grappled with seem to contradict common beliefs about black women's sexuality. Black hypersexuality and lasciviousness should have overwhelmed slave owners, not worries about black women's inability to reproduce fast enough.

Some enslaved women also held views that they could physically and mentally endure more physical pain than white women because of the condition of their enslavement. They were forced to do more work, swallow insults, and deal with absences from their loved ones, despair, and treatments for sicknesses overseen by white men. Leah Garrett remembered the audaciousness of a bondwoman who struck back at her white mistress for mistreatment and then ran away to live alone in a cave for years. As Leah recalled, the slave woman's husband formulated an escape plan, and the couple "lived in dis cave seven years."[37] To further embolden claims of the slave woman's resiliency and physical prowess, Leah commented that the woman had three children during her time in the cave. She stated, "Nobody was wid her when dese chillun was born but her husband. He waited on her wid each chile."[38] During childbirth, black mothers were supposedly unable to experience the "pain which attended women of the better classes."[39] While some enslaved women like Leah Garrett expounded on the strength of black women's bodies, slaves also noted black women's sensitivities in childbirth and postpartum recovery. The formerly enslaved Cato Carter remembered, "It was consid'ble hard on a woman when she had a frettin' baby."[40]

Frances Kemble, the famous English-born mistress of a large plantation in Georgia, kept a journal of the devastations enslaved women experienced when they became pregnant and gave birth. Kemble later chronicled the brutal conditions of slave lying-in hospitals. She wrote in her memoirs about the conditions of parturient enslaved women she observed over the course of one year, 1838–39: "These poor wretches lay prostrate on the earth . . . with no covering but the clothes they had on and some filthy rags of blanket."[41] She also described cases of two women who had undergone a "prolonged and terribly hard labor" with only an old black midwife to treat them.[42] The granny midwife served as "the sole matron, midwife, nurse, physician, surgeon, and servant of the infirmary."[43] The sickness and mortality rates in Kemble's slave hospital may have been high because of a practice that the enslaved caretaker used on her patients. She affixed "a cloth tight round the throats of the agonized women" and pulled it "till she almost suffocated them," which she believed aided in their labors.[44]

In extreme medical cases, white physicians explicitly described the sufferings of black women. In an 1835 article in the *American Journal of the Medical Sciences*, Dr. J. W. Heustis, of Mobile, Alabama, presented the case of an unidentified enslaved woman who suffered from a "strangulated umbilical hernia."[45] Although the physician described his slave patient as being in "extreme pain," he also wrote that her master described her recovery from surgery as "speedy."[46] In Heustis's example, the black female body might experience a serious ailment but could also heal more rapidly than other bodies. As some scholars of medicine and gender have noted, white physicians and slave owners found biblical support for their beliefs about the healing abilities of black women. The most commonly cited explanation concerning childbirth was the one centered on Eve, the first female character in the Christian creation story. She served as a spiritual reminder that God made women unequipped to manage birthing pain as punishment. Black women escaped the harsh pangs of labor because of an early interpretation of the "Hamitic curse" found in the Old Testament that misread Ham's children as being cursed with blackness.[47] Although women would want painless births, to have an easy childbirth, as black women were assumed to experience, would indicate that they escaped what was natural and biblically ordained for women after Eve's "fall." For some southern physicians, the Hamitic curse would demonstrate the accuracy of polygenism. Black women were not Eve's descendants and thus fell outside the scope of womanliness and pain related to childbirth. Despite polygenism's infamy in many southern medical circles, many southerners disagreed with the theory because of biblical contradictions. Many physicians, nonetheless, assumed that black women were innately "primordial" in nature.

Guiding the work of early surgeons was a dialectic that showed the sameness of the female anatomy. Despite conflicting racial and gender ideologies, the practice of medicine could specifically elucidate how ludicrous the era's racist science was, but doctors chose not to do so. As a slave owner, John Peter Mettauer believed in the inherent inferiority of black people, yet as a doctor, he experimented on bondwomen's bodies in hopes of curing all women of vesicovaginal fistula. Gender historian Sandra Harding offers her critique of this conundrum mired in racism and science, "Sexism, racism and class oppression construct and maintain each other, and they do this not once and for all, but over and over again in changing historical contexts. Both intentionally and unintentionally, they form mutual assistance bonds."[48]

Historian Marie Jenkins Schwartz has pointed out that bondwomen "found themselves struggling to control their own bodies."[49] Their actions were courageous because to assert ownership of oneself as a slave and a woman in antebellum America was contradictory to the law. For black women who were owned, their lives were forever guided by the landscape of American slavery, and for at least five decades, Irish immigrant women were defined by their racialized immigrant status. Despite their shared challenges, no matter how destitute and disempowered Irish-born women were in antebellum nineteenth-century America, enslaved women suffered worse fates because their blackness was inherent, not mapped onto them, and they were owned. As Jenkins Schwartz asserts, "society . . . did not define control of one's body as a fundamental right of slaves."[50]

African American anthropologist Zora Neale Hurston criticized the racial myopia of early twentieth-century publishing and offered an explanation for its willful ignorance of the complexities of nonwhite people: "The answer lies in what we may call the American Museum of Unnatural History. This is an intangible built on folk belief. It is assumed that all non-Anglo-Saxons are uncomplicated stereotypes. Everybody knows all about them. They are lay figures mounted in the museum where all may take them in at a glance. They are made of bent wires without insides at all."[51] Her critique is certainly applicable to analyzing how narrowly early American gynecologists conceived colored bodies in medicine and racial science. By pondering the analytical meaning of Hurston's metaphor of black bodies as mounted objects, we can recognize the deeply embedded racialized messages that are contained within and on Drana's naked body (see p. 87). Those men who pioneered gynecology treated enslaved black women like Drana as "mounted objects" devoid of complexity. With the inclusion of similarly disenfranchised Irish women in our historical treatment of their medical lives, we understand more fully that they were not simply objects to be read for study in medical texts and journals but were also complex subjects.[52]

Slavery, the making and remaking of blackness and otherness, and the defining and redefining the "female animal" made the contradictions of medical superbodies possible just as the social world of the nineteenth century could rely on black women held in medical bondage, all the while whitening them in the spaces where medical men could discuss freely how to handle black women's naked bodies. The presence and corresponding erasure of black women and poor Irish women reveals how the inner workings of the private medical sphere were constantly at odds with its public revelations. Thus black women could be praised for their fecundity in southern slavery, while poor Irish immigrant women could be demonized for birthing more children than they could care for in the northern cities where they lived. These women were linked to motherhood because they birthed children, not necessarily because Americans viewed poor Irish immigrant women as good mothers worthy of respect. Antebellumera America's rules on race, class, and gendered respectability did not allow these mothers to be lauded like the white medical men who experimented on their bodies. In this respect, gynecology would be no different. Black women and newly arrived immigrant women were always there to serve the interests of white physicians even while their bodies were broken or being mended.

The white medical gaze on black women's lives and bodies, the shifting scales on the continuum of racial sameness and difference, and white men's continued use of black women in gynecology were all grounded in ideas about black subjugation and white control. The black women bore the brunt of these ideas and practices all while coping with doctors' expectations that they would continue as laboring medical superbodies, performing the duties fit for a servant. The renewed interest in these women's medical lives provides greater insight into the history of slavery and medicine's development, the value of black and immigrant women to gynecology, and the importance of reassessing the place and value of historical actors in stories of origin.

AFTERWORD

·◖═══════════════◗·

O N A BEAUTIFUL AND UNSEASONABLY WARM DAY IN OCTOBER 2015, I
learned that I could not become pregnant naturally. As a result, I had to
have my cervix dilated so that my uterus would be more accessible for embryo
implantation during my initial in vitro fertilization procedure. The dilation was
conducted without my receiving either anesthesia or a numbing shot to ease
the pain. The doctor, one of the city's best fertility specialists, told me I would
experience some cramping but not a lot of pain. Pain was an understatement; I
had never gone through that kind of physical agony in my forty-three years of
life. The next month, the doctor dilated my cervix again without anesthesia. All
the while during the procedure, he kept apologizing for the pain he was causing
me. He even mentioned that he had thought to inject me with a numbing medi-
cation but decided against it since I had taken two Motrin pills. By New Year's
Day, I had changed physicians due to insurance issues. Also, I suspected that
if I brought my husband along with me to appointments, I would be perceived
differently by white doctors. I had to remind my previous doctor that I was
married, that, yes, my husband worked, although those questions stopped once
nurses and physicians saw my husband, a tall, physically imposing deep-voiced
man who is so light skinned that he looks like a white man.

My new specialist, a woman, was shocked when I informed her that I had
my cervix dilated without being given an anesthetic. Yet she also expressed
disbelief, after giving me a vaginal ultrasound, that my uterus was so small for
my body (it is not). I have small bones and am fewer than five feet six inches
tall; I assumed my uterus would not be especially large. It seemed that I could

not escape James Marion Sims's historical gaze but also the lessons he left for doctors who worked on the descendants of the original American "mothers of gynecology," held in medical bondage.

To theorize about nineteenth-century black women's bodies as medical superbodies impervious to pain is an exercise in analytical reasoning and historical methodology making. However, to live through a medical procedure in the twenty-first century in which the expectation was that I could tolerate acute pain seemed surreal. As I revealed to the medical staff during my dilation and hysterosalpingogram test (HSG), an X-ray test that looks at the inside of the uterus and fallopian tubes and the area around them, that I was writing a book about ideas about black women's bodies and pain thresholds, American gynecology, and James Marion Sims, my African American nurse stated, "Girl, you've got to tell your story too." My physician then shared with me how James Marion Sims pioneered fertility treatments in the United States. As I lay, contemplating their words and advice, I was struck by how time and space seemed to blur as the historical narrative of those women held in medical bondage in the 1840s was timely and important for black women who had to interact with present-day fertility specialists and gynecologists.

What my work as a historian of race, slavery, medicine, and gender has taught me is that the legacies from the nineteenth century are always present in our lives as Americans. I recognized that I was a benefactor of all the work that the country's earliest gynecologists performed on black women almost two hundred years prior. I had also inherited the burden that black women in the nineteenth century carried with them about their gynecological illnesses and the pain they felt: silence and dissemblance. Unlike the black women who helped to birth gynecology through their sufferings, I have a platform that allows me to reveal how black women still negotiate their lives as medical superbodies. From studies on black women as chronic pain sufferers who live with more pain than other Americans and have less access to pain-relief medicines to scholarship that highlights the ways that black gynecological patients have always had to deal with efforts to colonize their medical bodies, my own gynecological experiences in fertility medicine mirrored other black women's treatment.

I offer my medical experiences with fertility treatments for two reasons: I am a direct heir of James Marion Sims's medical legacy, and I reject critiques that demonize black and women scholars as unobjective when we dare to make personal connections with the historical actors we study, especially if they were enslaved. One of the better-known historical cases that center on objectivity, slavery, racism, and sexuality is the nearly two-decades-old controversy about

Thomas Jefferson's sexual relationship with Sally Hemings, his slave and his wife's younger half sister.

Not only did black scholars and the larger community believe the oral histories about Jefferson's affair, but they also disseminated the narrative. Black scholars knew that white southern slave owners impregnated enslaved women regularly on plantations and slave farms. Because of the lived experiences that African American scholars had as members of a racialized and historically marginalized group and their professional historical training, they were much more receptive to the idea that an elite and revered white man could maintain a sexual relationship with a much younger woman and keep her as his concubine. This combination of training and cultural socialization as an African American woman influenced me to read the sources differently for my book than had authors who had written previously about the birth of American gynecology and Dr. Sims. I suspected that if young enslaved women were being publicly exposed during the surgical procedures they endured over the years and were already assumed to be lascivious because they were black women, there might have been at least one birth on James Marion Sims's slave farm. Not only was I right, but also the baby was marked on the census record as a mulatto child.

As a twenty-first-century black gynecological patient, I was aware that my medical treatment might differ drastically from that of white women wishing to conceive. The specter of medical racism loomed because of the history of American women's medicine. Numerous medical studies have presented convincing evidence that African American women have more reproductive challenges than white women and experience racism and classism with their doctors.[1] The prospect of pregnancy seemed rooted in race as a biological construct no matter what I had been taught and accepted as a graduate student and later as a professor. All the doctors were white, and the nurses and ancillary staff were women of color. How could I not think of all things race-related when my blood work was sent to labs for genetic testing based on my "racial group"? Academics might have declared that race was a social construct, but doctors seemed to treat my blackness as biological. Although my work focuses on the antebellum era, the racial legacies of this period affect all Americans. Black women, the group that still represents the poorest Americans, the group that suffers from more reproductive ailments than other women in the country, and a demographic who mother as single women more than other American women are still being treated as superbodies in medicine. It is a sobering reality for me as I face my own battles reproductively despite my status as a married, educated, middle-class woman. Perhaps theorist Hortense Spillers was right: "I am a marked woman, but not everybody knows my name. . . . I describe a locus of confounded identities."[2] When I decided to write this book, I intended to not simply describe the racializing processes that created these clashing identities but to more accurately name and define them. So I went in search of the "mothers of gynecology"; in the process of my discoveries, I learned that I was their daughter, an already "marked woman."

NOTES

INTRODUCTION
AMERICAN GYNECOLOGY AND BLACK LIVES

1. Ivy, "Bodies of Work."

2. See Downs's *Sick from Freedom* and Samuel K. Roberts's *Infectious Fear.*

3. The non-Western humoral system was the Indian Ayurvedic one. The humoral system consisted of black bile, yellow bile, phlegm, and blood. It was widely accepted until the nineteenth century.

4. Willoughby, "Pedagogies of the Black Body," 4.

5. See Hartman's *Scenes of Subjection*, 58. Hartman investigates racial domination during slavery and how black people used terror and resistance to create identities.

6. My coining of the term "medical superbody" is inspired by Michele Wallace's black feminist book, *Black Macho and the Myth of the Superwoman.* The book examines the role of black women and their low status in American society.

7. O'Neill, *Five Bodies*, 123.

8. Ibid., 132.

9. Camp, *Closer to Freedom*, 8.

10. Walter Johnson, *Soul by Soul*, 136.

11. Gilman, "Black Bodies, White Bodies."

12. Stowe, *Doctoring the South*, 3.

13. See the work of historians such as the late Marli Weiner, Sharla Fett, Marie Jenkins Schwartz, and V. Lynn Kennedy for more information on the growing body of literature that focuses on slavery and histories of medicine.

14. Some of the secondary sources on Irish immigrant women were largely derived from Kuhn McGregor's *From Midwives to Medicine.*

15. See Bliss, *Blockley Days*; Dosite Postell, *Health of Slaves on Southern Plantations*; Emmet, *Reminiscences of the Founders*; Meigs, *Females and Their Diseases*; and Sims, *Story of My Life*.

16. Taylor, "Women in the Documents."

17. See Breeden, *Advice among Masters*.

18. Ibid., 164.

19. See Sandoval, *Methodology of the Oppressed*. This text positions love as a category of analysis, and I assert that a major component of the methodology of the oppressed born out of enslaved women's struggles is centered on the politicization of love.

20. Philips, *American Negro Slavery*.

21. Blassingame, *Slave Testimony*, 380.

22. Schroeder, *Slave to the Body*, 107.

23. Fanon, *Black Skin, White Masks*, 110.

CHAPTER I
THE BIRTH OF AMERICAN GYNECOLOGY

1. See Beverly, *History and Present State*.

2. Minges, *Far More Terrible for Women*, 183.

3. Ibid., 182.

4. Yetman, *Voices from Slavery*, 262.

5. See chap. 6, "The Masculine Birth of Gynaecology," in Monica H. Green's book *Making Women's Medicine Masculine* for a well-documented history of male midwifery and the rise of masculine authority in women's medicine during the fourteenth and fifteenth centuries, especially in Italy.

6. Walzer Leavitt, *Women and Health in America*, 149.

7. See Breeden's *Advice among Masters*.

8. Ebert, "Rise and Development," 243.

9. Ibid.

10. Ibid., 247.

11. Ibid., 260.

12. Sims, *Story of My Life*, 116.

13. Stephen Kenny, "Development of Medical Museums," 12.

14. Dain, *Hideous Monster of the Mind*, vii.

15. Walter Johnson, *Soul by Soul*, 136.

16. Gilman, "Black Bodies, White Bodies."

17. Spillers, "Mama's Baby, Papa's Maybe."

18. Eve and Meigs, "Article XII."

19. Pernick, *Calculus of Suffering*, 137.

20. Ibid.

21. Eve and Meigs, "Article XII," 395. Charles Meigs was one of America's most eminent medical doctors and professors of gynecology and obstetrics.

22. Schiebinger, *Nature's Body*, 160.

23. As early as the fourteenth century, adventurous European men had compiled popular travel narratives, such as *The Travels of Sir John Mandeville*, to introduce and discuss the differences of the people they allegedly encountered on their travels to Asia, Africa, and later the Americas. The author of this narrative expressed surprise at how comfortable black women were in displaying their nude bodies in front of both men and women. "Ethiopian [women]," he wrote, "have no shame of the men." See Morgan, *Laboring Women*, 16. "Bio-racism" is a more precise appellation for nineteenth-century racial theories than the more usual term "scientific racism."

24. Wood, *Origins of American Slavery*, 25.

25. Jefferson, *Notes on the State of Virginia*.

26. Ibid.

27. Contemporary scholars have termed this study of "science" pseudoscientific racism.

28. Gould, *Mismeasure of Man*.

29. Redpath, *Roving Editor*, 141.

30. Kuhn McGregor, *From Midwives to Medicine*, 111.

31. Brunton, *Women's Health and Medicine*, 51–52.

32. Caton, *What a Blessing*, 26.

33. See Breslaw's *Lotions, Potions, Pills, and Magic* for a discussion of the static nature of American medicine during the eighteenth and nineteenth centuries.

34. Rutkow, "Medical Education."

35. Waring, *History of Medicine*, 169.

36. All these surgeons began their work with both enslaved and white patient populations. Decades after this cohort of men transformed reproductive medicine, their colleagues termed them the "fathers" of various branches of American medicine.

37. Savitt, *Medicine and Slavery*, 293–97.

38. John Spurlock, "Vesicovaginal Fistula," *Medscape*, March 1, 2016, http://emedicine.medscape.com/article/267943-overview, accessed October 11, 2016.

39. Sims, *Story of My Life*, 241.

40. Wright, "On the Prussiate of Iron," 282–83.

41. Ibid., 282–83.

42. Ibid., 283. It is highly unlikely that the enslaved woman lost six pounds of blood. If she did in such a short period of time, the bondwoman would have gone into shock and died, because the human body contains only approximately six quarts, or twelve pounds, of blood. Wright must have miscalculated this amount.

43. Ibid.

44. Breslaw, *Lotions, Potions, Pills, and Magic*, 131.

45. Wright, "On the Prussiate of Iron," 280. While Dr. Wright did not state the race of the midwife, I believe she was white for several reasons, but mainly because she had access to prussiate of iron.

46. Ibid., 281. Prussian blue is the common name for prussiate of iron, because of its intense blue color. It is produced when ferrous ferrocyanide salts oxidize.

47. Ibid.

48. Weiner and Hough, *Sex, Sickness, and Slavery*, 43.

49. Archer, "Facts Illustrating a Disease," 319. The article does not provide information on the manner in which the women's labia were fused together. Dr. Archer's assertion that unsanitary conditions created the fusion of slave women's labia is misinformed. The numerous studies that contemporary scholars and researchers have authored about African retention practices and female genital mutilation provide a more accurate explanation of the origins of the bondwomen's condition. See Gomez's *Exchanging Our Country Marks* for a historical understanding of this kind of rite-of-passage practice.

50. Archer, "Facts Illustrating a Disease," 319.

51. Ibid.

52. Ibid.

53. Schachner, *Ephraim McDowell*, 131.

54. Young Ridenbaugh, *Biography of Ephraim McDowell*, 88.

55. Ibid., 88.

56. Nystrom, "Everyday Life in Danville." At the time 432 people lived in Danville, and most of those residents were white.

57. Johnston, *Sketch of Dr. John Peter Mettauer*, 9.

58. Mettauer, "On Vesico-Vaginal Fistula," 120.

59. Hartman, *Scenes of Subjection*, 85.

60. Sims, *Story of My Life*, 116.

61. Ibid., 32.

62. The seven articles that James Marion Sims published are listed in the order of their publication: "Double Congenital Harelip—Absence of the Superior Incisors, and Their Portion of Alveolar Process" (1844); "On the Extraction of Foreign Bodies from the Meatus Auditorius Externus" (1845); "Trismus Nascentium, Its Pathology and Treatment" (1846); "Removal of the Superior Maxilla for a Tumor of the Antrum. Apparent Cure. Return of the Disease. Second Operation. Sequel" (1847); "Osteo-Sarcoma of the Lower Jaw. Removal of the Body of the Bone without External Mutilation" (1847); "Further Observations of Trismus Nascentium, with Cases Illustrating Its Etiology and Treatment" (1848); and "On the Treatment of Vesico-Vaginal Fistula" (1852).

63. Sims, *Story of My Life*, 231.

64. Ibid., 227.

65. Ibid.

66. Ibid., 236.

67. Sims, *Silver Sutures in Surgery*, 52.

68. Ewell, *Medical Companion or Family Physician*, 46.

69. Dosite Postell, *Health of Slaves*, 138.

70. Douglass, "Brief Essay," 218.

71. Sims, *Story of My Life*, 237.

72. See Barker-Benfield, *Horrors of the Half-Known Life*.

73. Federal Census, Montgomery Ward, Montgomery, Alabama, December 5, 1850.

74. "Announcements."

75. See Harriet Washington's *Medical Apartheid*. Washington argues that pioneering doctors like James Marion Sims were intentionally racist and cruel in their treatment of enslaved women. While most white southern doctors who worked on black patients undoubtedly believed in their inferiority, it worked against the economic interests of slavery to willfully maim and murder black patients. All nineteenth-century medicine was experimental and exceedingly dangerous. Black women formed a more vulnerable patient population, as Washington argues, but the archival evidence does not point to white medical men behaving sadistically to devalue the medical lives of black women who kept slavery alive through their reproductive capabilities.

76. Rosenberg, *Care of Strangers*, 89.

77. Medical notes dated March 1853, William Darrach and George M. Darrach Papers, U.S. National Library of Medicine, National Institutes of Health, Bethesda, Md. Miss Manus may have informed the doctor that she was pregnant to gain medical treatment, especially if she was afraid of dying and leaving her children. Dropsy is a condition that causes severe swelling either in the body's cavities or in tissues.

CHAPTER 2

BLACK WOMEN'S EXPERIENCES IN SLAVERY AND MEDICINE

1. White men largely staffed the Works Progress Administration (WPA), developed by New Deal president Franklin Delano Roosevelt. Geneva Tonsill represented the small percentage of African American women who interviewed the formerly enslaved under the auspices of the WPA. Her presence was exceptional. Much has been written about how formerly enslaved men and women might have kowtowed to the often racially condescending treatment of white interviewers. Although scholars will never know the full extent of Julia Brown's honesty in responding to Geneva Tonsill's questions, we can reasonably guess that Brown might have felt a familiarity and community-linked kinship with an African American woman interviewer who was also living in a virulently racist Jim Crow America.

2. Yetman, *Voices from Slavery*, 48, and "Ex-Slave Interviews," 182.

3. *Arkansas Narratives*, 231.

4. *Athey v. Olive*, 34 Alabama 711 (1859), http://www.lib.auburn.edu/archive/aghy/slaves.htm, accessed March 25, 2015.

5. Dorothy Roberts, *Killing the Black Body*, 40.

6. Fett, *Working Cures*, 20.

7. Hurmence, *We Lived*, 100.

8. Jacobs, *Incidents in the Life*, 13.

9. Clayton, *Mother Wit*, 48.

10. Letter from William Lincrieux to Huger, July 3, 1847, Cleland Kinloch Huger Papers, South Caroliniana Library, University of South Carolina, Columbia.

11. Apter, "Blood of Mothers."

12. Ibid.

13. Schiebinger, *Nature's Body*, 160.

14. Archer, "Facts Illustrating a Disease," 320.

15. Ibid.

16. Bellinger, "Art. I.," 241–42.

17. Ibid., 242.

18. Ibid., 243.

19. Stephen N. Harris, "Case of Ovarian Pregnancy," 371–72.

20. Ibid., 372.

21. Ibid., 372. Contemporary physicians do not consider the use of iodide of potassium life threatening, although the risk for the developing goiters in utero for fetuses is increased. It is a pharmaceutical that iodizes salt and also aids in the treatment of thyroids.

22. Stephen N. Harris, "Case of Ovarian Pregnancy," 371–72.

23. Ibid., 372.

24. Tidyman, "Sketch," 337.

25. Weyers, *Abuse of Man*, 43.

26. Ibid.

27. Account Book, 1826, Frame 00154, John Peter Mettauer Papers, National Library of Medicine, National Institutes of Health, Bethesda, Maryland. Generally, white doctors charged twenty dollars for childbirth deliveries. The account book records kept by Joseph Mettauer document this fact. Mettauer visited "a negro woman in labour" at William Hynes's slave farm in November 1826 and was compensated this amount.

28. Redhibition is "the annulment of the sale of an article, etc., and its return to the vendor at the instigation of the buyer; (also) a civil action to compel a vendor to take back goods sold on the grounds of some defect." It is akin to contemporary "lemon laws." *Oxford English Dictionary*, 2016 online ed., s.v. "redhibition."

29. Tunnicliff Catterall, *Judicial Cases concerning American Slavery*, 2:320.

30. Ibid.

31. Ibid., 2:321.

32. Ibid.

33. Ibid., 2:331.

34. Pendelton, "Comparative Fecundity."

35. See Nell Irvin Painter's *Soul Murder and Slavery*. Painter defines "soul murder" as the system of brutality that affected the enslaved, especially children, who were sexually, emotionally, and physically abused by their owners. Drawing on psychiatry, Painter says that victims of "soul murder" quelled their emotions. She argues that soul murder was a regular feature of antebellum slavery, which was founded on severe violence.

36. Yetman, *Voices from Slavery*, 133.

37. Wyant Howell, *I Was a Slave*, 24–25.

38. Ibid., 25.

39. Williams, *Weren't No Good Times*, 78.

40. See Sharla Fett's *Working Cures*.

41. Yetman, *Voices from Slavery*, 47.

42. Eve and Meigs, "Article XII," 398.

43. Refers to Sharla Fett's 2002 book, *Working Cures*.

44. Yetman, *Voices from Slavery*, 230.

45. Dosite Postell, *Health of Slaves*, 118.

46. Tunnicliff Catterall, *Judicial Cases concerning American Slavery*, 2:672.

47. Ibid.

48. Ibid. Most notably, the court case mentions that the enslaved woman had no "delay and reluctance" in reporting her condition to her new owner, although her admission came on the fifteenth or twentieth of the month, a full twelve to seventeen days after he had acquired her.

49. Breslaw, *Lotions, Potions, Pills, and Magic*, 117.

50. The term "cachexia Africana" was coined by Samuel Cartwright, a founding member of the racist American school of ethnology. He first used the term in "Diseases and Peculiarities of the Negro Race" in *DeBow's Review*.

51. Harrison, "Cases in Midwifery," 369

52. Ibid.

53. Ibid., 369.

54. These two journals were used because they were the only two, as far as the research has revealed, that spanned over a twenty-year period, 1830–50. Nearly all nineteenth-century medical journals had very short publication lives.

55. The *Boston Medical and Surgical Journal* later became the *New England Journal of Medicine*, which is still in publication today.

56. If this enslaved woman was born in 1747, before the international slave trade ended, she quite possibly was born in West Africa. If so, she had more than likely participated in a female induction ceremony marking her transition from girlhood to womanhood. Though one can only speculate, she probably had a clitoridectomy performed on her while she was a young girl. After she was sold into slavery in America, the elderly enslaved woman had been removed from a distinct ethnic culture and society of women who could have at least offered her specific information on how to care for her body post-clitoridectomy and at the least, provide some methods, if they existed, of relieving her vaginal pain. To have her vagina mutilated as a young person and then to have a white male doctor manually examine her disfigured vagina with only his fingers must have been an unsettling emotional experience for the woman.

57. Bellinger, "Art. I," 248.

58. Ibid.

59. Ibid.

60. Copy of the Appraisement of the Personal Estate of Dr. James Spann, February 10, 1838, James Spann Papers, South Caroliniana Library, University of South Carolina, Columbia.

61. See the third chapter of Deborah Gray White's *Ar'n't I A Woman?*, 91–118. This chapter provides a detailed discussion of the evolution of female slaves' lives from childhood through their elderly years. Gray White also details the importance of reproduction and motherhood in these women's lives.

62. Harrison, "Cases in Midwifery," 367.

63. Ibid., 368.

64. Rawick, *American Slave*, 128.

65. Morris, *Culture of Pain*, 2.

66. Dorothy Roberts, *Killing the Black Body*, 42.

67. See Yetman, *Voices from Slavery*.

68. July was the birth month of three of the interviewees, or 11.11 percent of the total number.

69. There is a rich historiography on childbearing and enslaved women. See, for example, Cheryll Ann Cody's important article "Cycles of Work and of Childbearing: Seasonality in Women's Lives on Low Country Plantations." Cody writes, "Slave women in nonsugar areas . . . bore children in greater numbers, contributing, as in the case of the United States, to population growth" (in Gaspar and Clark Hine, *More Than Chattel*, 61). The author further argues that by looking at "the seasonality of labor in the fields and the seasonality of childbearing," scholars can assess how "annual cycles of crop production" were related to pregnancy and childbirth (62).

70. Gaillard, "Art. VII," 499.

71. "List of Negroes, 1844–1859," in Plantation Books, Glover Family Papers, South Caroliniana Library, University of South Carolina, Columbia. Also note that the literature on slave fertility helps to quantify the data on Glover Plantation slave births. As mentioned earlier, Cheryll Ann Cody's work on one thousand South Carolina bondwomen shows the linkages between a rather healthy diet and labor patterns and fertility rates. See Menken, Trussel, and Watkins's article "The Nutrition Fertility Link" for more information on the causative relationship between nutrition, labor, and fertility.

72. "List of Negroes, 1844–1859," Glover Family Papers.

73. "List of Negroes Sold, January 28, 1851," in Plantation Book, Glover Family Papers, South Caroliniana Library, University of South Carolina, Columbia.

74. "List of Inferior Negroes at Richfield Plantation, Belonging to Joseph and Edward Glover, 1852," in Plantation Book, Glover Family Papers, South Caroliniana Library, University of South Carolina, Columbia.

75. Blassingame, *Slave Testimony*, 380.

76. Ibid., 169.

77. Breeden, *Advice among Masters*, 169.

78. Woodman, *Slavery and the Southern Economy*, 89. For more information on the impact of intense labor during trimesters with resulting low birth weight, see Campbell, "Work, Pregnancy, and Infant Mortality."

79. Craghead, "Remarkable Case of Double Pregnancy," 114.

80. Breeden, *Advice among Masters*, 164.

81. Nordhoff, *Freedmen of South-Carolina*, 6

82. Hurmence, *Before Freedom*, 37.

83. Yetman, *Voices from Slavery*, 134.

84. Hurmence, *Before Freedom*, 79.

85. Medical Case Book (1860–1862), series/collection MC51, folder 246, J. J. A. Smith Papers, University of Alabama Archives, University of Alabama at Birmingham.

86. Hurmence, *Before Freedom*, 40.

87. Perdue, Barden, and Phillips, *Weevils in the Wheat*, 142.

88. Ibid. For another discussion of enslaved fatherhood, see Edward Baptist's "The Absent Subject."

89. Former slave Mary Reynolds's narrative, in *American Slave Narratives*.

90. Minges, *Far More Terrible for Women*, 26.

91. Alice Walker coined the term "womanism" in 1979 in her short story "Coming Apart." She grounded that theory in feminism and also the specific oppressive cultural, gendered, and racial realities that black women faced in American society.

92. Minges, *Far More Terrible for Women*, 26.

93. For more information, see Darlene Clark Hines groundbreaking article on black women, rape, and dissemblance, "Rape and the Inner Lives of Black Women in the Middle West."

CHAPTER 3
CONTESTED RELATIONS: SLAVERY, SEX, AND MEDICINE

1. Bailey, "Art. XI."

2. Ibid.

3. Ibid.

4. Peixotto, Rhinelander, and Graves, *New York Medical Journal*, 141.

5. Felstein, *Once a Slave*, 132. The following passage explains the consequences that some young black girls faced for being raped. "The mistress beat the child and locked her up in a smokehouse. For two weeks the girl was constantly whipped. Some of the elderly servants attempted to plead with the mistress on Maria's behalf, and even hinted that 'it was mass'r that was to blame.' The mistress's reply was typical: 'She'll know better in the future. After I've done with her, she'll never do the like again, through ignorance.'"

6. Bailey, "Art. XI."

7. Jacobs, *Incidents in the Life*, 55.

8. Ibid., 52.

9. Blassingame, *Slave Testimony*, 380.

10. Harrison, "Cases in Midwifery," 368.

11. Ibid.

12. *George (a slave) v. State*, 37 Miss 316, October 1859, p. 1249, Mississippi High Court of Errors and Appeals, Mississippi Supreme Court, *Mississippi State Cases: Being Criminal Cases Decided in the High Court of Errors and Appeals, and in the Supreme Court of the State of Mississippi: from the June Term 1818 to the First Monday in January 1872*, 1249.

13. See Melton, *Celia, a Slave*.

14. In *Without Consent or Contract*, Fogel writes extensively about the infant mortality rate of slave women in Trinidad and that of female slaves in the United States. Fogel

states, "In high-risk societies, some 60 percent of all infant deaths occurred within the first month following birth, nearly half of these early deaths occurred within hours, or at most a few days, after birth" (147–48). The period he references is circa 1830–50. White infant mortality rates in the antebellum South are nearly as grim as those of enslaved blacks according to Richard H. Steckel. He states, "The slave infant mortality rate calculated from plantation records in 233 per thousand. Approximately 201 of every thousand children who survived to age 1 did not survive to age 5. Although it is recognized that slave and white mortality rates may have differed, these data suggest that a figure in the neighborhood of 40 percent is not unreasonable." Steckel, "Antebellum Southern White Fertility," 336.

15. Block, *Rape and Sexual Power*, 100.

16. Dorothy Roberts, *Killing the Black Body*, 29–31.

17. Sommerville, *Rape and Race*, 265.

18. Fett, *Working Cures*, 11.

19. Wragg, "Article II," 146–47.

20. Ibid., 147.

21. Flexner, *Medical Education*, 3.

22. Savitt, *Race and Medicine*. Chapters 7 and 8 are especially vital to understanding the use of blacks in experimental surgeries and trials.

23. Dosite Postell, *Health of Slaves*, 118.

24. Walter Johnson's exhaustive study on the New Orleans antebellum slave markets, *Soul by Soul*, documents the medical examinations that slave women had to endure while being appraised by slave traders and merchants.

25. Finley, "Article V," 263.

26. Ibid. This enslaved woman may have had breast cancer, fibrocystic breasts, or a gynecological infection caused by a sexually transmitted disease.

27. Ibid., 264. Although not common, the practice of asking colleagues for help in locating the source of disease for medical cases was not exceedingly rare.

28. Ibid.

29. Hegel, *Phenomenology of Mind*, 235.

30. Wyant Howell, *I Was a Slave*, 28–29.

31. Ibid., 29.

32. Hill Collins, *Fighting Words*, 80.

33. Minges, *Far More Terrible for Women*, 183.

34. Williams, *Weren't No Good Times*, 111.

35. Hartman, *Scenes of Subjugation*, 81.

36. Camp, *Closer to Freedom*, 4.

37. Jordan, *White over Black*, 32.

38. Yetman, *Voices from Slavery*, 102–3.

39. Cott, *Bonds of Womanhood*, 187.

40. Williams, *Weren't No Good Times*, 78.

41. Atkins, "Atkins on the Rupture."

42. Brooks Higginbotham, "African American Women's History," 252.

43. Atkins, "Atkins on the Rupture," 332.

44. Jenkins Schwartz, *Birthing a Slave*, 3.

45. See Savitt, "Use of Blacks."

46. Perdue, Barden, and Phillips, *Weevils in the Wheat*, 142.

47. Historian Evelyn Brooks Higginbotham provides this definition and also adds that this supplanting of race by metalanguage makes it difficult to comprehend black women's lives and experiences.

48. Perdue, Barden, and Phillips, *Weevils in the Wheat*, 142.

49. Taylor, "Women in the Documents."

50. Dusinberre, *Them Dark Days*, 246–47.

51. Minges, *Far More Terrible for Women*, 153.

52. In the 1859 Louisiana judicial slave case of *Underwood v. Lacapère*, a slave owner sold a six-week-old boy along with his mother. The child had no listed value, and the bondwoman was undervalued at eight hundred dollars. The plaintiff indicated that the boy's presence "really diminished the then value of the mother." Taken from Helen Tunnicliff Catteral's *Judicial Cases concerning American Slavery*, 670. The sale of young infants negatively affected the economic value of their mothers because slave owners considered these totally dependent slaves financial burdens. Babies required monetary investments by slave masters and could not contribute to their owners' wealth until they were physically and mentally able to produce labor.

53. Minges, *Far More Terrible for Women*, 152–53.

54. Berlin, Favreau, and Miller, *Remembering Slavery*, 133.

55. Cott, *Bonds of Womanhood*, 193.

56. The theory of polygenism posits that human beings originated in different locations and are distinct in their biological and "racial" composition. Louis Agassiz was one of the earliest proponents of polygenism and wrote prolifically about the subject. He was one of the major proponents of the scientific racism that evolved in the nineteenth century.

57. The American school was developed by American physicians, ethnologists, and natural historians who claimed not only that races were distinct from one another but also that people of African descent were inherently inferior to those of European descent. The proponents of this biologically based racial science relied on craniometry and skeleton studies and the analysis of facial angles to determine how close black people were to apes.

CHAPTER 4
IRISH IMMIGRANT WOMEN AND AMERICAN GYNECOLOGY

1. "Destitute Emigrants."

2. Natalie Leger's comments from a September 19, 2015, writing group meeting, Brooklyn, New York. Also see Noel Ignatiev's *How the Irish Became White* and Hasia Diner's *Erin's Daughters in America*. For a discussion of the "othering" of the Irish by the English, see Audrey Horning's *Ireland in the Virginian Sea*.

3. Hassard, *Life of the Most Reverend John Hughes*, 309.

4. Ibid.

5. Dorsey, *Reforming Men and Women*, 195–240.

6. "The Missing Link," *Punch*, October 18, 1862, 165.

7. Maguire, *Irish in America*, 181.

8. Ibid., 340.

9. Fitzgerald, *Habits of Compassion*, 58.

10. Richardson, *History of the Sisters of Charity Hospital*, 2.

11. See chapter 2 of Maureen Fitzgerald's *Habits of Compassion*, esp. 73–76, for more detailed insight into the work of the House of the Good Shepherd and the contributions it made to the lives of Irish-born sex workers.

12. Ibid., 74.

13. Sanger, *History of Prostitution*, 594. In 1857, Blackwell Island burned, and Sanger's completed manuscript and personal library were lost to the fire. He had an original draft of his work that was finished in 1856, and he used this date to mark the completion of his writing and research although it was published years later.

14. Ibid., 594.

15. Charles E. Rosenberg, introduction, "Framing Disease: Illness, Society, and History," in Rosenberg and Golden, *Framing Disease*, xiv.

16. Sims, *Story of My Life*, 269. Although promoted as the country's first medical institution devoted solely to the treatment of gynecological diseases and ailments, Sims's Alabama slave hospital, in operation from 1845 to 1849, was the country's first women's hospital.

17. McCauley, *Who Shall Take Care of Our Sick?*, 3.

18. The appellation "Erin's Daughters" is derived from the Irish word for Ireland. Nineteenth-century poets and nationalists used it romantically to refer to Irish females. "Hibernia" was also a moniker for Irish women. See Diner, *Erin's Daughters in America*.

19. Rosenberg, *Care of Strangers*, 42.

20. Kuhn McGregor, *From Midwives to Medicine*, 105.

21. Ibid., 109.

22. Thomas Addis Emmet, although born in Virginia, was reared in New York. He did express sympathies with the South during the Civil War. Thus like some northerners because of either familial ties or cultural connections, he had a certain fondness for the South. Further, as a member of a famous Irish nationalist family, Emmet might not have discriminated against Mary Smith because of her Irish ancestry, but he was initially repulsed by her impoverished condition.

23. There is some speculation that James Marion Sims's southern sympathies, along with his practice of tightly packing medical theaters with onlookers, led to his being forced to leave the hospital he had founded right before the start of the Civil War.

24. Emmet, *Reminiscences of the Founders*, 5.

25. Kevin Kenny, *American Irish*, 107.

26. Gerber, *Making of an American Pluralism*, 130.

27. Niles, "Miscellaneous."

28. Takaki, *Iron Cages*, 116.

29. Lefkowitz Horowitz, *Rereading Sex*, 9.

30. Kevin Kenny, *American Irish*, 63.

31. Information on the history of the House of Industry in South Boston can be accessed at the Harvard Business School in Cambridge, Mass. The electronic library record is available at http://www.library.hbs.edu/hc/wes/indexes/alpha/content/1001955798.html, accessed December 21, 2007.

32. Jackson, "Malformation," 394.

33. Dexter, "Singular Case of Hiccough," 195.

34. Ibid., 196.

35. Ibid.

36. Ibid.

37. Ibid., 197.

38. Ibid.

39. Rosenberg, *Framing Diseases*, xvi.

40. Löwy, "Historiography of Biomedicine."

41. Meigs, *Lecture*, 5.

42. Kraut, *Silent Travelers*, 41.

43. Burnwell, "Article IV," 323.

44. Ibid.

45. Thomas, *History of Nine Cases*, 11.

46. Fitzgerald, *Habits of Compassion*, 83.

47. Elliot, "Induction of Premature Labor," 331.

48. Fordos, "On the Employment," 206.

49. Elliot, "Induction of Premature Labor," 333.

50. Ibid.

51. Gliddon and Nott, "Types of Mankind."

52. Churchill, "Observations on the Diseases."

53. Thomas, *History of Nine Cases*, 5.

54. Ibid., 6.

55. Gegan, "Case of Spontaneous Rupture," 360.

56. Ibid.

57. Ibid., 361.

58. Ibid.

59. Ibid.

60. Ibid.

61. Ibid., 362.

62. Agnew, "Vesico-Vaginal Fistula," 572.

63. Ibid.

64. Ibid.

65. Ibid.

66. According to the Saint Joseph Hospital's website, "in 1849, Ireland was experiencing a devastating famine, which sent people fleeing to the United States. For Irish immigrants who settled in Philadelphia, medical attention was desperately needed. To

answer the growing medical needs of these immigrants, a substantial three-story home at the corner of Sixteenth Street and Girard Avenue was purchased. This dwelling would soon come to be known as Saint Joseph's Hospital, the oldest Catholic hospital in the city of Philadelphia." http://www.nphs.com/stjo_info.html.

67. Agnew, "Vesico-Vaginal Fistula," 572.

68. Irish women's bodies and facial features were drawn to resemble apes throughout the century. For a more critical discussion of the history of the simianization of the Irish, see Curtis, *Apes and Angels* and *Anglo-Saxons and Celts*. Roy Porter also writes about simianization and anti-Irish racism in his book *Paddy and Mr. Punch*. The names "Paddy" and "Mr. Punch" refer to the stereotypical and also animal-like representations of the Irish that were found in British humor periodicals and literature. See also Laura Briggs's "The Race of Hysteria."

69. Briggs, "Race of Hysteria," 262.

70. MS B 324, William Darrach and George M. Darrach Papers, History of Medicine Division, National Library of Medicine, U.S. National Institutes of Health, Bethesda, Md.

71. Warner, *Popular Treatise*, 109.

CHAPTER 5
HISTORICAL BLACK SUPERBODIES AND THE MEDICAL GAZE

1. Sims, *Story of My Life*, 470–71.

2. Morrison, *Race-ing Justice, En-gendering Power*, xi.

3. Curran, *Anatomy of Blackness*, 223–24.

4. Anne Fausto-Sterling, "Gender, Race, and Nation: The Comparative Anatomy of 'Hottentot' Women in Europe, 1815–17," in Wallace-Sanders, *Skin Deep, Spirit Strong*, 72.

5. Schiebinger, *Nature's Body*, 135.

6. Fields and Fields, *Racecraft*, 17.

7. Brooks Higginbotham, "African-American Women's History," 252.

8. Schiebinger, *Nature's Body*, 156.

9. Breeden, *Advice among Masters*, 164.

10. Cartwright, "Diseases and Peculiarities."

11. Sims, *Story of My Life*, 228–29.

12. Ibid., 230.

13. Ibid.

14. Ibid., 238.

15. Curran, *Anatomy of Blackness*, 224.

16. Sims, *Story of My Life*, 242.

17. Curtis, *Apes and Angels*, 12.

18. Ibid., 13.

19. Jordan, *White over Black*, 238.

20. Walzer Leavitt, *Women and Health in America*, 13.

21. Ibid., 12.

22. Meigs, *Females and Their Diseases*, 46–47.

23. Nell Irvin Painter notes the importance of Johann Friedrich Blumenbach as "The Father of Anthropology" and as "a Founding Father of racial science and the classification of races." More information about the relevance of Blumenbach's work within racial science can be found in Irvin Painter's unpublished essay, "Why Are White People Called 'Caucasian'?"

24. Schiebinger, *Nature's Body*, 163.

25. Ibid.

26. Gallaher, "Case of Rupture," 291.

27. *Code of Ethics*, 5.

28. Ibid., 7 and 9.

29. Archer, "Facts Illustrating a Disease," 323.

30. Stephanie M. H. Camp, "The Pleasures of Resistance: Enslaved Women and Body Politics in the Plantation South, 1830–1861," in Baptist and Camp, *New Studies in the History*, 93. Camp defines the "outlawed body" as a "site of pleasure and resistance" for an enslaved person. Further, she sees the outlawed body as a "third body . . . and a political site."

31. Archer, "Facts Illustrating a Disease," 323.

32. For further information on Archer, consult the biographical article by J. Alexis Shriver, "Dr. John Archer."

33. Archer, "Facts Illustrating a Disease," 323.

34. Wyant Howell, *I Was a Slave*, 15.

35. See Wyant Howell, *I Was a Slave*. Laura Clark, who was formerly held in bondage, responded in her WPA interview that her "mammy was de mother of twenty-two chillun," while Lulu Wilson reported that she was her parents' only child. Due to Wilson's only-child status, her mother was forced to "marry" another man, and they produced "nineteen chillen."

36. Wyant Howell, *"I Was a Slave,"* 33.

37. Minges, *Far More Terrible for Women*, 22.

38. Ibid., 22.

39. Pernick, *Calculus of Suffering*, 156.

40. Wyant Howell, *"I Was a Slave,"* 33.

41. Kemble, *Journal of a Residence*, 363–64.

42. Ibid.

43. Ibid.

44. Ibid.

45. Heustis, "Case of Strangulated Umbilical Hernia," 380.

46. Ibid., 381.

47. Noted American school physician and proslavery racist Samuel Cartwright gave a "scientific" explanation for black people's biological defects as they related to Ham. Cartwright wrote, "The verb, from which his Hebrew name is derived, points out this flexed position of his knees, and also clearly expresses the servile type of his mind. Ham, the father of Canaan, . . . a black man was the father of the slave or knee-bending

species of mankind. . . . The Negro, in all ages of the world, has carried with him a mark equally efficient . . . the mark of blackness." Samuel Cartwright, "The Prognathous Species of Mankind," in McKitrick, *Slavery Defended*, 143.

48. Harding, "Taking Responsibility," 14.

49. Jenkins Schwartz, *Birthing a Slave*, 3.

50. Ibid., 3.

51. Hurston, "What White Publishers Won't Print."

52. Portions of this chapter appear in my chapter "Perfecting the Degraded Body: Slavery, Irish-Immigration, and American Gynaecology," in *Power in History: From Medieval Ireland to the Post-Modern World*, ed. Anthony McElligott, Liam Chambers, Ciara Breathnach, and Catherine Lawless (Dublin: Irish Academic Press, 2011).

AFTERWORD

1. Dr. Desiree McCarthy-Keith, an African American endocrinologist, has found that "11.5% of black women report infertility compared to 7% of white women . . . yet studies indicate that black women use infertility services less often." Georgia Reproductive Specialists, "African American Women and Infertility: An Unmet Need," *PR Newswire*, April 2, 2012, http://www.prnewswire.com/news-releases/african-american-women-and-infertility-an-unmet-need-145776205.html.

2. Spillers, "Mama's Baby, Papa's Maybe," 65.

BIBLIOGRAPHY

MANUSCRIPT AND ARCHIVAL SOURCES

John Black Papers. South Caroliniana Library, University of South Carolina, Columbia, South Carolina.

William Darrach and George M. Darrach Papers. U.S. National Library of Medicine, National Institute of Health, Bethesda, Maryland.

Glenn Drayton Papers. South Caroliniana Library, University of South Carolina, Columbia, South Carolina.

Edward and William Glover Family Papers. South Caroliniana Library, University of South Carolina, Columbia, South Carolina.

Cleland Kinloch Huger Papers. South Caroliniana Library, University of South Carolina, Columbia, South Carolina.

John Peter Mettauer Papers. U.S. National Library of Medicine. National Institutes of Health, Bethesda, Maryland.

J. J. A. Smith Papers. University of Alabama Archives. Reynolds-Finley Historical Library, University of Alabama at Birmingham, Alabama.

James Spann Papers. South Caroliniana Library, University of South Carolina, Columbia, South Carolina.

James Davis Trezevant Papers. South Caroliniana Library, University of South Carolina, Columbia, South Carolina.

NEWSPAPERS AND MAGAZINES

Charleston Courier, 1837
Cork Examiner, 1848
Medical News, 1848

New York Times, 1851–65
Punch, 1862

MEDICAL JOURNALS

Baltimore Medical and Philosophical Lycaeum
Boston Medical and Surgical Journal
Carolina Journal of Medicine, Science and Agriculture
Charleston Medical Journal and Review
DeBow's Review of the Southern and Western States. Devoted to Commerce, Agriculture, Manufactures
Journal of American Medical Sciences
Journal of the American Medical Association
Louisville Journal of Medicine and Surgery
Medical and Surgical Reporter
Medical Examiner
Medical Examiner and Record of Medical Science
Medical News
Medical Repository of Original Essays and Intelligence, Relative to Physic, Surgery, Chemistry, and Natural History
New York Medical Journal
North American Medical and Surgical Journal
Philadelphia Journal of Medical and Physical Sciences
Southern Journal of Medicine and Pharmacy
Virginia Medical Monthly

GOVERNMENT RECORDS

Federal Census, Montgomery Ward, Montgomery, Alabama, December 5, 1850.
United States Census Bureau. "Resident Population and Apportionment of the U.S. House of Representatives." http://www.census.gov/dmd/www/resapport /states/kentucky.pdf.

PUBLISHED PRIMARY SOURCES

Agnew, D. Hayes. "Vesico-Vaginal Fistula," *Medical and Surgical Reporter* 6, no. 26 (September 1861): 572–73.
American Slave Narratives: An Online Anthology. http://xroads.virginia.edu/~hyper /wpa/reynold1.html.
"Announcements." *Medical News* 6, no. 65. (May 1848): 60.
Archer, John. "Facts Illustrating a Disease Peculiar to the Female Children of Negro Slaves, and Observations, Showing That a White Woman by Intercourse with a White Man and a Negro, May Conceive Twins, One of Which Shall Be White, and the Other a Mulatto; and That, Vice Versa, a Black Woman by Intercourse with a Negro and a White Man, May Conceive Twins, One of Which Shall be a Negro and the Other a Mulatto." *Medical Repository of Original Essays and Intel-*

ligence, *Relative to Physic, Surgery, Chemistry, and Natural History* 1 (February–April 1810): 319–23.

Arkansas Narratives. Vol. 2, pt. 3 of *Slave Narratives: A Folk History of Slavery in the United States from Interviews with Former Slaves*. Typewritten Records Prepared by the Federal Writers' Project, 1936–1938. Assembled by the Library of Congress Project Works Project Administration for the District of Columbia. Sponsored by the Library of Congress, Washington, D.C., 1941. http://memory .loc.gov/mss/mesn/023/023.pdf.

Atkins, Charles. "Atkins on the Rupture of the Uterus and Vagina, Terminating in Recovery, with Remarks on These Accidents." *Carolina Journal of Medicine, Science and Agriculture* 1, no. 3 (July 1825): 332–42.

Bailey, R. S. "Art. XI.—Case of Rape.—Death the Consequence," *Charleston Medical Journal and Review* 6, no. 1 (January 1851): 676.

Baldwin, William O. "Observations on the Poisonous Properties of the Sulphate of Quinine," *American Journal of Medical Sciences* 13, no. 26 (April 1847): 292–310.

Beecher, Catharine. *Letters to the People on Health and Happiness*. New York: Harper & Brothers, 1855.

Bellinger, John. "Art. I.—Operations for the Removal of Abdominal Tumours. Case I.—Extirpation of an Ovarian Tumour, Complicated with Hydrops Uteri—Recovery." *Southern Journal of Medicine and Pharmacy* 2, no. 3. (May 1847): 241–45.

Beverly, Robert, Jr. *The History and Present State of Virginia*. 1705, 1722. http://natio nalhumanitiescenter.org/pds/becomingamer/growth/text1/virginiabeverley.pdf.

Bliss, Arthur Ames. *Blockley Days: Memories and Impressions of a Resident Physician, 1883–1884*. Philadelphia: Printed for private distribution, 1916.

Buell, W. P. "Report on the Diseases of Females Treated at the New York Dispensary, from May 1842 to May 1843." *American Journal of Medical Sciences* 7, no. 13 (January 1844): 96–117.

Burnwell, George N. "Article IV.—Statistics and Cases of Midwifery; Compiled from the Records of the Philadelphia Hospital, Blockley." *American Journal of the Medical Sciences* 7, no. 14 (April 1844): 317–39.

Campbell, Henry F., and Robert Campbell. *Regulations of Jackson Street Hospital, and Surgical Infirmary for Negroes*. Augusta, Ga.: Jeremiah Morris, Printer, 1859. http://archive.org/stream/regulationsoojack/regulationsoojack_djvu.txt.

Cartwright, Samuel. "Agricultural and Plantation Department: Diseases and Peculiarities of the Negro Race." *DeBow's Review of the Southern and Western States. Devoted to Commerce, Agriculture, Manufactures* 1, no. 1. (July 1851): 64–74.

Churchill, Fleetwood. "Observations on the Diseases Incident to Pregnancy and Childbed." *Boston Medical and Surgical Journal* (1840): 250.

"City Poor—Interesting Items of Number, Cost, & c.—New Plan of Supporting Them, & c." *Journal of Prison Discipline and Philanthropy* 14, no. 1 (January 1859): 22–26.

Code of Ethics of the American Medical Association. Philadelphia: T. K. & P. G. Collins, 1854.

Craghead, William G. "A Remarkable Case of Double Pregnancy—One Ovum Entering the Uterus, the Other Being Arrested in the Tube. Communicated by Hugh L. Hodge, M.D., Professor Midwifery in the University of Pennsylvania." *American Journal of the Medical Sciences* 19, no. 37 (January 1850): 114–16.

"Destitute Emigrants." In *The Ocean Plague by a Cabin Passenger*, 118–23. Boston: n.p., 1848. Reprinted from the *Cork Examiner*

Dexter, George T. "Singular Case of Hiccough Caused by Masturbation." *Boston Medical and Surgical Journal* 32, no. 10 (April 1845): 195–97.

Douglass, John. "A Brief Essay on the Best Mode of Preserving Health on Plantations." *Southern Journal of Medicine and Pharmacy* 2, no. 1. (February 1847): 216–19.

Dunbar, Paul Laurence. *Lyrics of Lowly Life*. London: Chapman & Hall, 1897.

Elliot, George T. "Induction of Premature Labor with the Douche." *New York Journal of Medicine* 2, no. 3 (May 1857): 331.

Emmet, Thomas Addis. *Incidents of My Life, Professional, Literary, Social, with Services in the Cause of Ireland*. New York: G. P. Putnam's Sons, Knickerbocker Press, 1911.

———. *Reminiscences of the Founders of the Woman's Hospital Association*. New York: Stuyvesant Press, 1893.

Eve, Paul F., and Charles D. Meigs. "Article XII—Case of Excision of the Uterus." *American Journal of Medical Sciences* (October 1850): 40, 397.

Ewell, James. *The Medical Companion or Family Physician*. Philadelphia: Carey, Lea, & Blanchard, 1834.

Fenner, C. S. "Vesico-Vaginal Fistula." *American Journal of the Medical Sciences* 38, no. 76 (October 1859): 353–55.

Finley, S. B. R. "Article V.—Case of Menstruation from the Mammae." *Carolina Journal of Medicine, Science, and Agriculture* 1, no. 3 (July 1825): 263–64.

Fordos, M. "On the Employment of Carbonic Acid as a Medicinal Agent." In *The Retrospect of Practical Medicine and Surgery*, edited by W. Braithwaite, 205–8. New York: W. A. Townsend, 1859.

Fox, George. "Article I. Account of a Case in Which the Cæsarean Section, Performed by Prof. Gibson, was a Second Time Successful in Saving Both Mother and Child." *American Journal of Medical Sciences* 22, no. 43 (May 1838): 13–23.

———. "Midwifery." *North American Medical and Surgical Journal* 12, no. 24 (October 1831): 484–92.

Gaillard, P. C. "Art. VII.—Remarks on Trismus Nascentium." *Southern Journal of Medicine and Pharmacy* 1, no. 1 (January 1846): 499–506.

Gallaher, Thomas J. "Case of Rupture of the Uterus." *Medical Examiner and Record of Medical Science* 14, no. 77 (May 1851): 291–95.

Gegan, John, Jr. "Case of Spontaneous Rupture of the Uterus." *Medical and Surgical Reporter* 1, no. 21 (February 1859): 360–62.

Gliddon, George, and Josiah Nott. "Types of Mankind." *Georgia Blister and Critic* 1, no. 5 (July 1854): 112.

Hamilton, George. "Case of Diseased Uterus." *Medical Examiner* 3, no. 10 (March 1840): 157–58.

Harris, Stephen N. "Case of Ovarian Pregnancy." *Southern Journal of Medicine and Pharmacy* 1, no. 1 (January 1846): 371–77.

Harris, William Lett. "John Peter Mettauer, A.M., M.D., LL.D.: A Country Surgeon." *American Medical Association*. Reprinted from the *Virginia Medical Monthly* (November 1926): 1–18.

Harrison, John P. G. "Cases in Midwifery." *American Journal of the Medical Sciences* 15, no. 30 (February 1835): 366–74.

Hassard, John R. G. *Life of the Most Reverend John Hughes, D.D, First Archbishop of New York, with Extracts from His Private Correspondence*. New York: D. Appleton, 1866.

Hegel, Georg Wilhelm Friedrich. *The Phenomenology of Mind*. Translated with an introduction and notes by J. B. Baillie. London: G. Allen & Unwin; New York: Humanities Press, 1931.

Heustis, J. W. "Case of Strangulated Umbilical Hernia, with Removal of the Cyst, Followed by a Radical Cure." *American Journal of the Medical Sciences* 26, no. 32 (August 1835): 380–81.

Jackson, J. B. S. "Malformation of the Internal Genital Organs in an Adult Female." *American Journal of Medical Sciences* 22, no. 44 (August 1838): 393–95.

Jacobs, Harriet. *Incidents in the Life of a Slave Girl*. 1861; repr., New York: Oxford University Press, 1988.

Jarvis, Edward. "Insanity among the Coloured Population of the Free States: Table I. Table II. Table III. Table IV. Deaf and Dumb and Blind, among the Coloured Population." *American Journal of the Medical Sciences* 7, no. 13. (January 1844): 71–84.

Jefferson, Thomas. *Notes on the State of Virginia*. 1782; repr., Boston: Lilly & Wait, 1832.

Johnson, Charles S. *Shadow of the Plantation*. http://www.dollsgen.com/slavenarratives.html.

Johnston, George Ben. *A Sketch of Dr. John Peter Mettauer of Virginia*. Richmond, Va.: American Surgical Association, 1905.

Kelly, Howard. *Medical Gynecology*. New York: D. Appleton, 1908.

Kemble, Frances. *Journal of a Residence on a Georgian Plantation in 1838–1839*. New York: Harpers & Brothers, Franklin Square, 1863.

Maguire, John Francis. *The Irish in America*. London: Longmans, Green, 1868.

Meigs, Charles D. *Females and Their Diseases: A Series of Letters to His Class*. Philadelphia: Lea & Blanchard, 1848.

———. *Lecture on Some of the Distinctive Characteristics of the Female, Delivered before the Class of the Jefferson Medical College*, Philadelphia, January 5, 1847. Philadelphia: T. K. and P. G. Collins, Printers, 1847.

Mettauer, John Peter. "Vesico-Vaginal Fistula." *Boston Medical and Surgical Journal* 22, no. 10 (April 1840): 154–55.

————. "On Vesico-Vaginal Fistula." *American Journal of Medical Sciences* 14, no. 27 (July 1847): 117–21.

Niles, Hezekiah. "Miscellaneous." *Niles Weekly Register*, November 2, 1834, 132.

Nordhoff, Charles. *The Freedmen of South-Carolina: Some Account of Their Appearance, Character, Condition, and Peculiar Customs*. New York: Charles T. Evans, 1863.

"On The Diseases Incident to Pregnancy and Child-bed." *Boston Medical and Surgical Journal* 23, no. 16 (November 1840): 1–8.

Pendelton, E. M. "The Comparative Fecundity of the Black and White Races." *Charleston Medical Journal and Review* 6 (1851): 351.

Redpath, James. *The Roving Editor; or, Talks with Slaves in Southern States*. New York: A. B. Burdick, 1859.

Sanger, William W. *The History of Prostitution: Its Extent, Causes, and Effects throughout the World*. New York: Harper, 1859.

Savage, Henry. *The Surgery, Surgical Pathology, and Surgical Anatomy of the Female Pelvic Organs, in a Series of Coloured Plates Taken from Nature* (London: John Churchill & Sons, 1862).

Sims, James Marion. *Silver Sutures in Surgery: The Anniversary Discourse before the New York Academy of Medicine*. New York: Samuel S. & William Wood, 1858.

————. *The Story of My Life*. New York: D. Appleton, 1884.

————. "Trismus Nascentium—Its Pathology and Treatment." *American Journal of the Medical Sciences* 11, no. 21 (April 1846): 363–81.

Small, E. *A Treatise on Inflammatory Disease of the Uterus, and Its Appendages, and on Ulceration and Enlargement of the Neck of the Uterus in Which the Morbid Uterine Manifestations and Functional Derangements Are Explained and Illustrated*. Boston: Sanborn, Carter & Bazin, 1856.

Stevens, Alex H. "A Case of Contraction to the Vagina, from Sloughing Caused by a Tedious Labour in Which the Cicatrix Was Safely Divided by a Bistourie to Facilitate Parturition during a Subsequent Labour." *Medical and Surgical Register, Consisting Chiefly of Cases in the New York* 1, pt. 2 (June 1820): 163–70.

Swett, John A. "Protracted Adhesion of a Portion of the Placenta, with Final Sloughing." *Boston Medical and Surgical Journal* 13, no. 14 (November 1835): 217–19.

Thomas, T. Gaillard. *The History of Nine Cases of Ovariotomy*. New York: D. Appleton, 1869.

Tidyman, Philip G. "Sketch of the Most Remarkable Diseases of the Negroes of the Southern States with an Account of the Method of Treating Them, Accompanied by Physiologic Observations." *Philadelphia Journal of Medical and Physical Sciences* 3, no. 6 (April 1826): 306–38.

Tiedemann, Frederick. "On the Brain of the Negro, Compared with That of the European and the Ourang-Outang." *Louisville Journal of Medicine and Surgery* 1, no. 1 (January 1838): 245–46.

Tunnicliff Catterall, Helen, ed. *Judicial Cases concerning American Slavery and the Negro*. Vol. 2, *Cases from the Courts of North Carolina, South Carolina, and Tennessee*. Washington, D.C.: Carnegie Institution of Washington, 1929.

Visiting Committee Minutes. Massachusetts General Hospital Association. March 23, 1827.

Warner, Lucien. *A Popular Treatise on the Functions and Diseases of Women.* New York: Manhattan, 1874.

Whyte, Robert H. *The Journey of an Irish Coffin Ship,* http://xroads.virginia.edu /~HYPER/SADLIER/IRISH/RWhyte.htm, from *The Ocean Plague; or, A Voyage to Quebec in an Irish Immigrant Vessel* (Boston: Coolidge and Wiley, 1848).

Wragg, John A. "Article II.—Case of Rupture of the Uterus." *Southern Journal of Medicine and Pharmacy* 2, no. 1 (March 1847): 146–48.

Wright, Thomas H. "On the Prussiate of Iron in Uterine Hemorrhage." *Baltimore Medical and Philosophical Lycaeum* 1, no. 3 (July 1811): 279–83.

SECONDARY SOURCES

"African American Women and Infertility: An Unmet Need." PRNewswire. http:// www.prnewswire.com/news-releases/african-american-women-and-infertility -an-unmet-need-145776205.html.

Anbinder, Tyler. "From Famine to Five Points: Lord Lansdowne's Irish Tenants Encounter North America's Most Notorious Slum." *American Historical Review* 107, no. 2 (April 2002): 351–87.

Apter, Andrew. "The Blood of Mothers: Women, Money, and Markets in Yoruba-Atlantic Perspective." *Journal of African American History* 98, no. 1 (Winter 2013): 72-98.

Baptist, Edward. "The Absent Subject: African-American Masculinity and Forced Migration to the Antebellum Plantation Frontier." In *Southern Manhood: Perspectives on Masculinity in the Old South.* Athens: University of Georgia Press, 2004.

Baptist, Edward E., and Stephanie M. H. Camp. *New Studies in the History of American Slavery.* Athens: University of Georgia Press, 2006.

Barker-Benfield, G. J. *The Horrors of the Half-Known Life: Male Attitudes toward Women and Sexuality in Nineteenth-Century America.* New York: Harper & Row, 1976.

Berlin, Ira, Marc Favreau, and Steven F. Miller, eds. *Remembering Slavery: African Americans Talk about Their Personal Experiences of Slavery and Freedom.* New York: New Press in association with the Library of Congress, 1998.

Blakely, Robert, and Judith Harrington. *Bones in the Basement: Postmortem Racism in Nineteenth-Century Medical Training.* Washington, D.C.: Smithsonian Institute Press, 1997.

Blassingame, John W., ed. *Slave Testimony: Two Centuries of Letters, Speeches, Interviews, and Autobiographies.* Baton Rouge: Louisiana State University Press, 1977.

Block, Sharon. *Rape and Sexual Power in Early America.* Chapel Hill: University of North Carolina Press, 2006.

Breeden, James O., ed. *Advice among Masters: The Ideal in Slave Management in the Old South.* Westport, Conn.: Greenwood Press, 1980.

Breslaw, Elaine G. *Lotions, Potions, Pills, and Magic: Health Care in Early America.* New York: New York University Press, 2012.

Briggs, Laura. "The Race of Hysteria: 'Overcivilization' and the 'Savage' Woman in Late Nineteenth-Century Obstetrics and Gynecology." *American Quarterly* 52, no. 2. (June 2000): 246–73.

Brooks Higginbotham, Evelyn. "African American Women's History and the Meta-language of Race." *Signs* 17, no. 2 (Winter 1992): 251–74.

Brunton, Deborah. *Women's Health and Medicine: Health and Wellness in the Nineteenth Century*. Santa Barbara, Calif.: Greenwood Press, 2014.

Byrd, W. Michael, and Linda A. Clayton. *An American Health Dilemma: A Medical History of African Americans and the Problems of Race; Beginnings to 1900*. New York: Routledge, 2000.

Camp, Stephanie M. H. *Closer to Freedom: Enslaved Women and Everyday Resistance in the Plantation South*. Chapel Hill: University of North Carolina Press, 2004.

———. "The Pleasures of Resistance: Enslaved Women and Body Politics in the Plantation South, 1830–1861." *Journal of Southern History* 68, no. 3 (August 2002): 533–72.

Campbell, John. "Work, Pregnancy, and Infant Mortality among Southern Slaves." *Journal of Interdisciplinary History* 14, no. 4 (Spring 1984): 793–812.

Caton, Donald. *What a Blessing She Had Chloroform: The Medical and Social Response to the Pain of Childbirth from 1800 to the Present*. New Haven, Conn.: Yale University Press, 1999.

Clark Hine, Darlene. *HineSight: Black Women and the Re-Construction of American History*. Brooklyn: Carlson, 1994.

———. "Rape and the Inner Lives of Black Women in the Middle West: Preliminary Thoughts on the Culture of Dissemblance." Special issue, "Common Grounds and Crossroads: Race, Ethnicity, and Class in Women's Lives," *Signs* 14, no. 4 (Summer 1989): 912–20.

Clark Hine, Darlene, and Kathleen Thompson. *A Shining Thread of Hope: The History of Black Women in America*. New York: Broadway Books, 1998.

Clayton, Ronnie. *Mother Wit: The Ex-slave Narratives of the Louisiana Writers' Project*. New York: Peter Lang, 1990.

Cooper Owens, Deirdre B. "The Tie That Binds: Black and Irish Women's Bodies, Experimental Surgery and Reproductive Care." Paper presented at the Ninety-Second Annual Association for the Study of African-American Life and History, Charlotte, N.C., October 2007.

Cott, Nancy F. *The Bonds of Womanhood: "Women's Sphere" in New England, 1780–1835*. 2nd ed. New Haven, Conn.: Yale University Press, 1997.

———, ed. *Root of Bitterness: Documents of the Social History of American Women*. New York: E. P. Dutton, 1972.

Curran, Andrew S. *The Anatomy of Blackness: Science and Slavery in an Age of Enlightenment*. Baltimore: Johns Hopkins University Press, 2013.

Curtis, L. Perry, Jr. *Anglo-Saxons and Celts: A Study of Anti-Irish Prejudice in Victorian England*. Bridgeport, Conn: Conference on British Studies at the University of Bridgeport, 1968. Distributed by New York University Press.

————. *Apes and Angels: The Irishman in Victorian Caricature*. Washington, D.C.: Smithsonian Institution Press, 1997.

Dain, Bruce. *A Hideous Monster of the Mind: American Race Theory in the Early Republic*. Cambridge, Mass.: Harvard University Press, 2002.

Dezell, Maureen. *Irish America: Coming into Clover; The Evolution of a People and a Culture*. New York: Doubleday, 2000.

Diner, Hasia R. *Erin's Daughters in America: Irish Immigrant Women in the Nineteenth Century*. Baltimore: Johns Hopkins University Press, 1983.

Dooley, Brian. *Black and Green: The Fight for Civil Rights in Northern Ireland and Black America*. London: Pluto Press, 1998.

Dorsey, Bruce. *Reforming Men and Women: Gender in the Antebellum City*. Ithaca, N.Y.: Cornell University Press, 2002.

Dosite Postell, William. *The Health of Slaves on Southern Plantations*. Baton Rouge: Louisiana State University Press, 1951.

Downs, Jim. *Sick from Freedom: African-American Illness and Suffering during the Civil War and Reconstruction*. New York: Oxford University Press, 2012.

Doyle, Bertram Wilbur. *The Etiquette of Race Relations in the South: A Study in Social Control*. Chicago: University of Chicago Press, 1937.

Dusinberre, William. *Them Dark Days: Slavery in the American Rice Swamp*. New York: Oxford University Press, 1996.

Ebert, Myrl. "The Rise and Development of the American Medical Periodical 1797–1850." *Journal of Medical Library Association* 100, E (July 1952): 243–76.

Eltis, David. "Europe, Revolution and the Transatlantic Slave Trade." Paper presented to the History Department at the University of California, Los Angeles, November 8, 2007.

Fanon, Frantz. *Black Skin, White Masks*. Translated by Charles Lam Markmann. New York: Grove Press, 1967.

Felstein, Stanley, ed. *Once a Slave: The Slaves' View of Slavery*. New York: William Morrow, 1971.

Fett, Sharla. *Working Cures: Healing, Health, and Power on Southern Slave Plantations*. Chapel Hill: University of North Carolina Press, 2002.

Fields, Barbara, and Karen E. Fields. *Racecraft: The Soul of Inequality in American Life*. London: Verso, 2012.

Finkelman, Paul. *Slavery and the Founders: Race and Liberty in the Age of Jefferson*. Armonk, N.Y.: M. E. Sharpe, 2001.

Fitzgerald, Maureen. *Habits of Compassion: Irish Catholic Nuns and the Origins of New York's Welfare System, 1830–1920*. Urbana: University of Illinois Press, 2006.

Flexner, Abraham. *Medical Education in the United States and Canada: A Report to the Carnegie Foundation for the Advancement of Teaching*. Bulletin no. 4. New York: Carnegie Foundation for the Advancement of Teaching, 1910.

Fogel, Robert William. *Without Consent or Contract: The Rise and Fall of American Slavery*. New York: Norton, 1989.

Gaspar, David Barry, and Darlene Clark Hine. *More Than Chattel: Black Women and Slavery in the Americas.* Bloomington: Indiana University Press, 1996.

Geary, Laurence M. *Medicine and Charity in Ireland, 1718–1851.* Dublin: University College Dublin Press, 2004.

Genovese, Eugene. *The Political Economy of Slavery: Studies in the Economy and Society of the Slave South.* New York: Pantheon Books, 1965.

Gentile O'Donnell, Donna. *Provider of Last Resort: The Story of the Closure of the Philadelphia General Hospital.* Philadelphia: Camino Books, 1995.

Gerber, David. *The Making of an American Pluralism: Buffalo, New York, 1825–60.* Urbana: University of Illinois Press, 1989.

Gilman, Sander L. "Black Bodies, White Bodies: Toward an Iconography of Female Sexuality in Late-Nineteenth-Century Art, Medicine, and Literature." *Critical Inquiry* 12, no. 1 (Autumn 1985): 204–42.

Gomez, Michael. *Exchanging Our Country Marks: The Transformation of African Identity in the Colonial and Antebellum South, 1526–1830.* Chapel Hill: University of North Carolina Press, 1998.

Gould, Steven Jay. *The Flamingo's Smile.* New York: Norton, 1985.

———. *The Mismeasure of Man.* New York: Norton, 1996.

Graham Goodson, Martha. "Enslaved Africans and Doctors in South Carolina." *Journal of the National Medical Association* 95, no. 3 (March 2003): 225–33.

Gray, Laman A. *The Life and Times of Ephraim McDowell.* Louisville, Ky.: Gheens Foundation, 1987.

Gray White, Deborah. *Ar'n't I a Woman? Female Slaves in the Plantation South.* New York: Norton, 1985.

Green, Monica H. *Making Women's Medicine Masculine: The Rise of Male Authority in Pre-modern Gynecology.* Oxford: Oxford University Press, 2008.

Groneman, Carol. "Working-Class Immigrant Women in Mid-Nineteenth-Century New York: The Irish Woman's Experience." *Journal of Urban History* 4, no. 3 (May 1978): 255–73.

Harding, Sandra. "Taking Responsibility for Our Own Gender, Race, Class: Transforming Science and the Social Studies of Science." *Rethinking Marxism* 11, no. 3 (Fall 1989): 8–19.

Harris, Leslie M. *In the Shadow of Slavery: African Americans in New York City, 1626–1863.* Chicago: University of Chicago Press, 2003.

Hartman, Saidiya V. *Scenes of Subjugation: Terror, Slavery, and Self-Making in Nineteenth-Century America.* New York: Oxford University Press, 1997.

Hill Collins, Patricia. *Black Feminist Thought: Knowledge, Consciousness, and the Politics of Empowerment.* 2nd ed. New York: Routledge, 2000.

———. *Fighting Words: Black Women and the Search for Justice.* Minneapolis: University of Minnesota Press, 1998.

Horning, Audrey. *Ireland in the Virginian Sea: Colonialism in the British Atlantic.* Chapel Hill: University of North Carolina Press. 2014.

Hurmence, Belinda, ed. *Before Freedom, When I Just Can Remember: Twenty-Seven Oral Histories of Former South Carolina Slaves.* Winston-Salem, N.C.: John F. Blair, 1989.

———. *We Lived in a Little Cabin in the Yard.* Winston-Salem, N.C.: John F. Blair, 1994.

Hurston, Zora Neale. "What White Publishers Won't Print." *Negro Digest*, April 1950, 89.

Ignatiev, Noel. *How the Irish Became White.* New York: Routledge, 1995.

Irvin Painter, Nell. "Why White People Are Called 'Caucasian.'" Paper presented at the Fifth Annual Gilder Lehrman Center International Conference, for the "Collective Degradation: Slavery and the Construction of Race" panel, Yale University, New Haven, Conn., November 8, 2003.

Ivy, Nicole. "Bodies of Work: A Meditation on Medical Imaginaries and Enslaved Women." *Souls: A Critical Journal of Black Politics, Society, and Culture* 18, no.1 (June 2016): 11–31.

James, Joy, and T. Denean Sharpley-Whiting. *Black Feminist Reader.* Malden, Mass.: Blackwell, 2000.

Jenkins Schwartz, Marie. *Birthing a Slave: Motherhood and Medicine in the Antebellum South.* Cambridge, Mass.: Harvard University Press, 2006.

Johnson, Walter. *Soul by Soul: Life inside the Antebellum Slave Market.* Cambridge, Mass.: Harvard University Press, 1999.

Jones, Jacqueline. *Labor of Love, Labor of Sorrow: Black Women, Work, and the Family from Slavery to the Present.* New York: Basic Books, 1985.

Jordan, Winthrop D. *White over Black: American Attitudes toward the Negro, 1550–1812.* Chapel Hill: University of North Carolina Press, 1968.

Kenny, Kevin. *The American Irish: A History.* Essex, U.K.: Pearson Education Limited, 2000.

Kenny, Stephen. "The Development of Medical Museums in the Antebellum American South: Slave Bodies in Networks of Anatomical Exchange." *Bulletin of the History of Medicine* 87, no. 1 (Spring 2013): 12.

Kerber, Linda K., Alice Kessler-Harris, and Kathryn Kish Sklar. *U.S. History as Women's History: New Feminist Essays.* Chapel Hill: University of North Carolina Press, 1995.

Kraut, Alan M. *Silent Travelers: Germs, Genes, and the "Immigrant Menace."* Baltimore: Johns Hopkins University Press, 1995.

Kuhn McGregor, Deborah. *From Midwives to Medicine: The Birth of American Gynecology.* New Brunswick, N.J.: Rutgers University Press, 1998.

Lefkowitz Horowitz, Helen. *Rereading Sex: Battles over Sexual Knowledge and Suppression in Nineteenth-Century America.* New York: Vintage Books, 2002.

Löwy, Ilana. "Historiography of Biomedicine: 'Bio,' 'Medicine,' and In Between." *Isis* 102, no. 1 (March 2011).

Lucas, Marion B. *A History of Blacks in Kentucky: From Slavery to Segregation, 1760–1891.* Lexington: University Press of Kentucky, 2003.

Lynch-Brennan, Margaret. "Ubiquitous Biddy: Irish Immigrant Women in Domestic Service in America, 1840–1930." PhD diss., University at Albany, State University of New York, 2002.

"Marion Sims and the Southern Gynecologists." *Journal of the American Medical Association* 60, no. 4. (January 1913): 285.

McCaffrey, Lawrence J. *The Irish Diaspora in America.* Washington, D.C.: Catholic University of America Press, 1984.

McCauley, Bernadette. *Who Shall Take Care of Our Sick? Roman Catholic Sisters and the Development of Catholic Hospitals in New York City.* Baltimore: Johns Hopkins University Press, 2005.

McElligott, Anthony, Liam Chambers, Ciara Breathnach, and Catherine Lawless. *Power in History: From Medieval Ireland to the Post-Modern World.* Dublin: Irish Academic Press, 2011.

McKitrick, Eric L. *Slavery Defended: The Views of the Old South.* Englewood Cliffs, N.J.: Prentice-Hall, 1963.

Melton, Robert, ed. *Celia, a Slave.* Athens: University of Georgia Press, 1991.

Menken, Jane, James Trussel, and Susan Watkins. "The Nutrition Fertility Link: An Evaluation of the Evidence." *Journal of Interdisciplinary History* 11, no. 3 (Winter 1981): 425–44.

Minges, Patrick, ed. *Far More Terrible for Women: Personal Accounts of Women in Slavery.* Winston-Salem, N.C.: John F. Blair, 2006.

Morantz-Sanchez, Regina. *Conduct Unbecoming a Woman: Medicine on Trial in Turn-of-the-Century Brooklyn.* New York: Oxford University Press, 1999.

Morgan, Jennifer. *Laboring Women: Reproduction and Gender in New World Slavery.* Philadelphia: University of Pennsylvania Press, 2004.

Morris, David B. *The Culture of Pain.* Berkeley: University of California Press, 1991.

Morrison, Toni, ed. *Race-ing Justice, En-gendering Power: Essays on Anita Hill, Clarence Thomas, and the Construction of Social Reality.* New York: Pantheon Books, 1992.

Numbers, Ronald, and Todd L. Savitt. *Science and Medicine in the Old South.* Baton Rouge: Louisiana State University Press, 1989.

Nystrom, Judy. "Everyday Life in Danville during Dr. Ephraim McDowell's Era, 1802–1830". Washington, D.C.: American College of Obstetricians and Gynecologists, 1989.

O'Neill, John. *Five Bodies: The Human Shape of Modern Society.* Ithaca, N.Y.: Cornell University Press, 1985.

Painter, Nell Irvin. *Soul Murder and Slavery: Toward a Fully Loaded Cost Accounting.* Waco, Tex.: Baylor University Press, 1995.

Perdue, Charles L., Thomas E. Barden, and Robert K. Phillips, eds. *Weevils in the Wheat: Interviews with Virginia Ex-slaves.* Charlottesville: University Press of Virginia, 1976.

Pernick, Martin S. *A Calculus of Suffering: Pain, Professionalism, and Anesthesia in Nineteenth-Century America.* New York: Columbia University Press, 1985.

Philips, Ulrich B. *American Negro Slavery: A Survey of the Supply, Employment, and Control of Negro Labor, as Determined by the Plantation Regime*. New York: D. Appleton, 1918.

Porter, Roy. *Paddy and Mr. Punch: Connections in Irish and English History*. London: Allen Lane, 1993.

Rawick, George P., ed. *The American Slave: A Composite Autobiography*. Westport, Conn.: Greenwood, 1972.

Richardson, Jean. *A History of the Sisters of Charity Hospital, Buffalo, New York, 1848–1900*. Lewiston, N.Y.: Edwin Mellen Press, 2005.

Roberts, Dorothy. *Killing the Black Body: Race, Reproduction, and the Meaning of Liberty*. New York: Vintage Books, 1997.

Roberts, Samuel K. *Infectious Fear: Politics, Disease, and the Health Effects of Segregation*. Chapel Hill: University of North Carolina Press, 2009.

Roediger, David. *The Wages of Whiteness: Race and the Making of the American Working Class*. London: Verso, 1991.

Rosenberg, Charles E. *The Care of Strangers: The Rise of America's Hospital System*. Baltimore: Johns Hopkins University Press, 1987.

Rosenberg, Charles E., and Janet Golden, eds. *Framing Disease: Studies in Cultural History*. New Brunswick, N.J.: Rutgers University Press, 1991.

Rutkow, Ira M. "Medical Education in Early 19th Century America." *Archives of Surgery* 134, no. 4 (April 1999): 453.

Sandoval, Chela. *Methodology of the Oppressed: Theory out of Bounds*. Minneapolis: University of Minnesota Press, 2000.

Sappol, Michael. *A Traffic of Dead Bodies: Anatomy and Embodied Social Identity in Nineteenth-Century America*. Princeton, N.J.: Princeton University Press, 2002.

Savitt, Todd L. *Medicine and Slavery: The Diseases and Health Care of Blacks in Antebellum Virginia*. Urbana: University of Illinois Press, 1978.

———. *Race and Medicine in Nineteenth- and Early-Twentieth-Century America*. Kent, Ohio: Kent State University Press, 2007.

———. "The Use of Blacks for Medical Experimentation and Demonstration in the Old South." *Journal of Southern History* 48, no. 3 (August 1982): 331–48.

Schachner, August. *Ephraim McDowell: "Father of Ovariotomy" and Founder of Abdominal Surgery, with an Appendix on Jane Todd Crawford*. Philadelphia: J. B. Lippincott, 1921.

Schiebinger, Londa. *Nature's Body: Gender in the Making of Modern Science*. Boston: Beacon Press, 2004.

Schroeder, Lars. *Slave to the Body: Black Bodies, White No-Bodies and the Regulative Dualism of Body-Politics in the Old South*. Frankfurt: Peter Lang, 2003.

Shriver, Alexis J. "Dr. John Archer: The First Graduate of Medicine in America (1768), and His Home 'Medical Hall,' in Harford County, Maryland." *Bulletin of the Medical Library Association* 20, no. 3 (January 1932): 90–101.

Sommerville, Diane Miller. *Rape and Race in the Nineteenth-Century South*. Chapel Hill: University of North Carolina Press, 2004.

Spillers, Hortense. "Mama's Baby, Papa's Maybe: An American Grammar Book," *Diacritics* 17, no. 2 (Summer 1987): 64–81.

Steckel, Richard H. "Antebellum Southern White Fertility: A Demographic and Economic Analysis." *Journal of Economic History* 40, no. 2 (June 1980): 331–50.

Stevenson, Brenda E. *Life in Black and White: Family and Community in the Slave South.* New York: Oxford University Press, 1996.

Stowe, Steven M. *Doctoring the South: Southern Physicians and Everyday Medicine in the Mid-Nineteenth Century.* Chapel Hill: University of North Carolina Press, 2004.

Takaki, Ronald. *Iron Cages: Race and Culture in Nineteenth-Century America.* New York: Oxford University Press, 1990.

Taylor, Ula. "Women in the Documents: Thoughts on Uncovering the Personal, Political, and Professional." *Journal of Women's History* 20, no. 1 (Spring 2008): 187–96.

Walker, Alice. *In Search of Our Mothers' Gardens: Prose.* San Diego: Harcourt Brace Jovanovich, 1983.

Wallace, Michele. *Black Macho and the Myth of the Superwoman.* New York: Dial Press, 1979.

Wallace-Sanders, Kimberly. *Skin Deep, Spirit Strong: The Black Female Body in American Culture.* Malden, Mass.: Blackwell, 2000.

Walter, Bronwen. *Outsiders Inside: Whiteness, Place, and Irish Women.* London: Routledge, 2001.

Walzer Leavitt, Judith. *Brought to Bed: Childbearing in America, 1750–1950.* New York: Oxford University Press, 1988.

———. *Women and Health in America: Historical Readings.* Madison: University of Wisconsin Press, 1984.

Waring, Joseph. *A History of Medicine in South Carolina, 1670–1825.* Vol. 1. Columbia: South Carolina Medical Association, 1964.

Washington, Harriet. *Medical Apartheid: The Dark History of Medical Experimentation on Black Americans from Colonial Times to the Present.* New York: Doubleday, 2007.

Weiner, Marli. *Mistresses and Slaves: Plantation Women in South Carolina, 1830–80.* Urbana: University of Illinois Press, 1997.

Weiner, Marli, and Mazie Hough. *Sex, Sickness, and Slavery: Illness in the Antebellum South.* Urbana: University of Illinois Press, 2012.

Weyers, Wolfgang. *The Abuse of Man: An Illustrated History of Dubious Medical Experimentation.* New York: Ardor Scribendi, 2003.

Williams, Horace Randall, ed. *Weren't No Good Times: Personal Accounts of Slavery in Alabama.* Winston-Salem, N.C.: John F. Blair, 2004.

Willoughby, Christopher. "Pedagogies of the Black Body: Race and Medical Education in the Antebellum United States." PhD diss., Tulane University, 2016.

Wood, Betty. *The Origins of American Slavery: Freedom and Bondage in the English Colonies.* New York: Hill & Wang, 1997.

Woodman, Harold D. *Slavery and the Southern Economy: Sources and Readings*. New York: Harcourt, Brace & World, 1966.

Wyant Howell, Donna, ed. *I Was a Slave: True Life Stories Told by Former American Slaves in the 1930s*. Washington, D.C.: American Legacy Books, 1997.

Yancy, George. *White Gazes: The Continuing Significance of Race*. Lanham, Md.: Rowman & Littlefield, 2008

Yetman, Norman. "Ex-Slave Interviews and the Historiography of Slavery," *American Quarterly* 36, no. 2 (1984): 181–210.

———. *Life under the "Peculiar Institution": Selections from the Slave Narrative Collection*. New York: Holt, Rinehart & Winston, 1970.

———. *Voices from Slavery: 100 Authentic Slave Narratives*. Mineola, N.Y.: Dover, 1999.

Young Ridenbaugh, Mary. *The Biography of Ephraim McDowell, M.D.: "The Father of Ovariotomy."* New York: Charles L. Webster, 1890.

INDEX

abortion, 41, 66, 71, 73, 87

African people, 21–22, 116, 129n23; ape relation, 114–15; cultural practices, 45–46

Agassiz, Louis, 87, 137n56

agency, 34, 44, 48, 71; acts of resistance, 81–82, 85; pregnancy or reproductive, 58, 70, 85, 105

Agnew, Dr. D. Hayes, 105–6

American Journal of Medical Sciences (*AJMS*), 34, 39, 76, 98, 119, 133n54; articles on sexual surgeries, 55

American Medical Association (AMA), 18–19, 20, 41, 102; Code of Ethics, 116; establishment and purpose, 26, 51

American medicine, 9, 18, 84; criticisms, 31–32; ethics, 47–48, 102, 116; experimental nature of, 42, 51; female conditions and, 115; professionalization of, 26; prominent medical men, 25, 129n36; roots of, 5–6. *See also* gynecology; medical journals; reproductive medicine

anesthesia, 11, 24, 96, 123

ape-human link, 82, 94, 106, 114–15, 140n68

Apter, Andrew, 45

Archer, Dr. John, 29–30, 46, 53, 116–17, 130n49

Athey, Henry, 43

Athey v. Olive, 43

Atkins, Dr. Charles, 10, 83, 84

autonomy. *See* agency

Bailey, Dr. R. S., 73–74

Beaumont, William, 48

Bellinger, Dr. John, 55–56

biological difference: of black and white women, 8, 17, 21, 28, 84, 107, 111; polygenism theory of, 87, 137n56; among races, 103, 106–7, 137n5

bio-racism, 100, 129n23. *See also* scientific racism

Black Codes, 106

blackness, 21, 41, 50, 107, 120; biblical interpretation of, 119, 141n47; concept of, 109; cultural production of, 27; doctors' views of, 53; mapped on to Irish women, 20, 88, 95; race and biology and, 2, 4, 5–6, 23, 110, 125

black scholars, 124–25

black women: bodies, 6–7, 10, 19, 21, 54, 108–9, 129n23; as "breeders," 19–20, 38, 50, 84, 118; elderly, 56, 133n56; exceptionalization of, 21; as impervious to pain, 21, 44, 108, 110–12, 114, 118–19, 123–24; medical experiences of, 41, 42–44; metanarratives of, 83–87; methodology of oppressed and, 10–11, 128n19; as

CPSIA information can be obtained
at www.ICGtesting.com
Printed in the USA
LVHW091754031120
670609LV00007B/674